Occupation –

Of every kind – however varied, requires to be alternated, fairly, with rest & recreation –

Strictly, no occupation that calls forth special mental & physical work should fill more than 1/3 of the daily life. The body of man is not constructed to run its completed cycle under a heavier burden of labour

Sleep – 8 hours – best if an [illegible] procedure between 10 & 6 – Room to be well ventilated.

Bath – sponge – [illegible] 24 hours –

Water is the only natural beverage

# HUMPHREYS'

# HOMEOPATHIC MENTOR

OR

## FAMILY ADVISER

IN THE USE OF

## SPECIFIC HOMEOPATHIC MEDICINE.

BY

F. HUMPHREYS, M. D.,

Late Professor of Institutes of Homeopathy, Pathology and Medical Practice in the Homeopathic Medical College of Pennsylvania at Philadelphia: Author of Dysentery and its Homeopathic Treatment; Cholera and its Homeopathic Treatment; and Prover of Apis Mellifica, Plantago Major, etc., etc.

---

NEW YORK:
HUMPHREYS' SPECIFIC HOMEOPATHIC MEDICINE CO.,
562 BROADWAY.
1874.

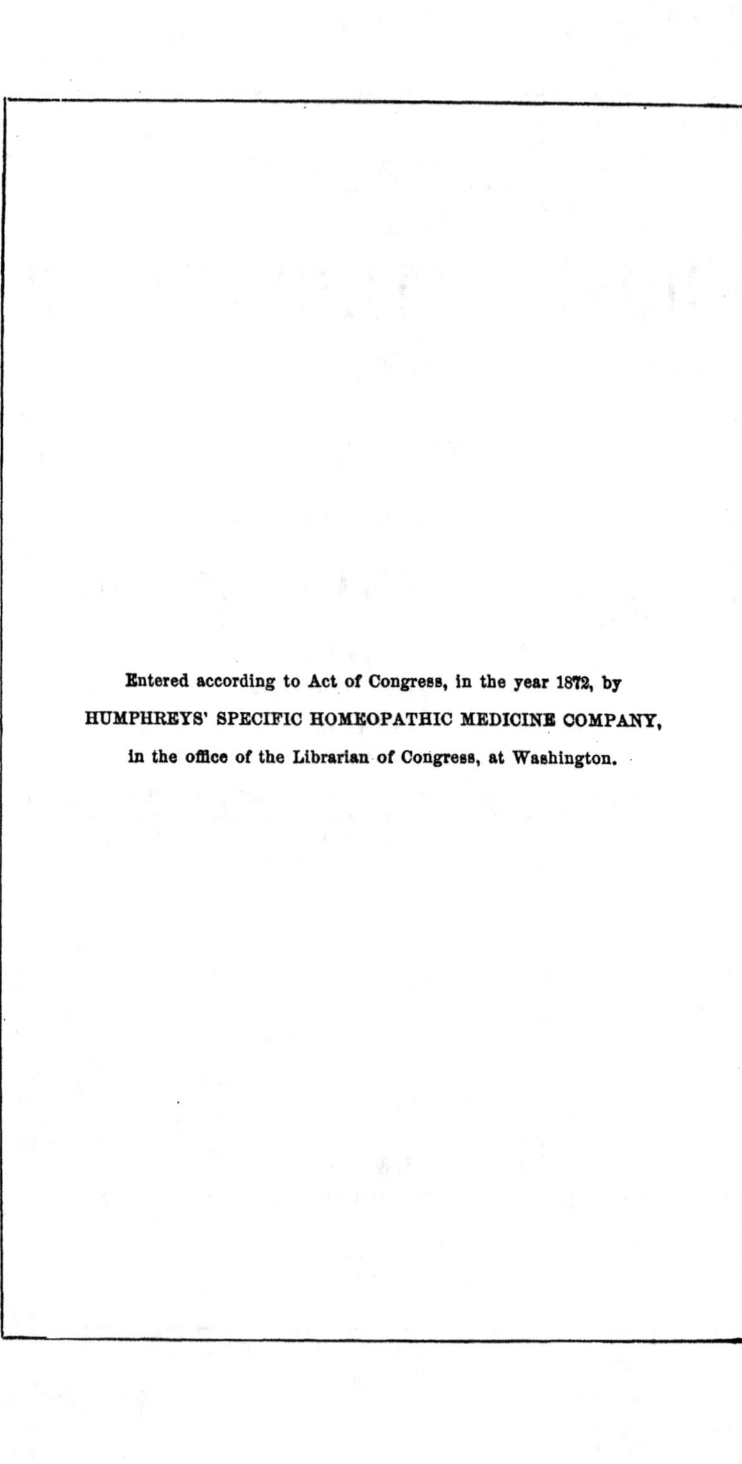

Disease of Kidney fr. Alcohol

Excessive indulgence of malt liquors is a common cause of calculus -

Alcohol very soon gives rise to unnatural renal secretions - to a fine deposit of pinkish sedimentary matter - & occasional production of a fine film of fatty or iridescent substance on the surface of the fluid after standing. This is the condition favorable to Calculus

Alcoholic dyspepsia -

Stomach & alimentary canal surcharged with gases flatulence

depression of mind & ready irritation.

Action of bowels irregular - now constipated now relaxed.

Urine now copious & pale -
now scanty - loaded with pink deposit
Coated with fine fatty like iridescent film or pellicle. -

Sleep irregular. -

Disease from sloth -

Ennui - hypochondriacal fancies dread of death, despondency & despair suggesting suicide

Feeble resistance to cold - succumb under slight attacks of disease - premature old age -

Tempted to eat too much, hence a feeble heart, weakened vascular mechanism of brain - syncope, apoplexy

They know nothing of true happiness - for life with inactivity is a physical burden

The indolent heart passes into unnatural forms of motion. the sluggish brain is reconstructed out of devitalized material - hence organic degeneration, & premature death from failure of vascular or nervous power

Mental feebleness, imbecility - Doubt - hesitation, distrust, fear despondency & despair -

# PREFACE.

It is now twenty years since I commenced the experimentation and use of Specific or Combined Homeopathic Medicines, the results of which, in a popular, practical form, I now present in this work. I have waited long, perhaps too long, that I might not be accused of rashly offering crude or immature views; and yet, remembering how little, comparatively, one man can do in so wide a field, in even so long a period, I could wish the time longer, and the experience more ample. If it shall lead to greater precision in the use of medicine, and a more complete control over human disease and suffering, my labor will have been amply rewarded. The snatches of time for its production, taken from the exactions of large professional and business cares, must apologize for any want of unity or defects of style that may appear in its composition.

The theme is new. Old-school medicines have been compounded or combined for centuries, and Polypharmacy has been the rule, as well as the opprobrium of its practitioners. The rule of Hahnemann was exact and rigorous—one medicine, in its highest attenuation, given once, and permitted, undisturbed, to expend its action—formed the ideal of Homeopathic practice. To this rule, the professor and the amateur, the adept and the satellite, were expected to conform. The choice of the medicine was to be made, not so much according to the physiological or pathological similia, as according to some *key note,* or fantastic aberration, alike of medicine and disease, the study of which was a psychological phantasmagoria.

But practical men, and practical medicine, with too little, perhaps, of faith, and too little, certainly, of result, unwilling to attribute all failure to the bluntness of their own perceptions, hesitating to follow the shadow of the master, when their footsteps so often fell on dead men's bones, turned aside to seek more substantial footing in larger doses, frequent repetitions, and alternation of remedies. The success becomes as sure, the labor less, and the way plainer. But what becomes of the ideal Hahnemannean rule—the one medicine, the one dose, and undisturbed action? It is buried in a sea, so deep, as to be practically fathomless.

But what becomes of the similia, the law of cure, when modes so different, paths so apparently divergent, lead to the same goal? Simply this: THE LAW OF CURE IS WIDER THAN WE KNOW. Not to so narrow channels as we have believed, are the waters of this Bethesda confined. Simple and childlike may his faith be, who believes that in his hands alone, is the cup of healing; a deeper knowledge and wider experience would have placed it in the hands of others as well.

From alternated to combined medicines (Specifics) the transition is easy. The old rule of faith and practice is gone. A wider field is opened and we are invited to enter. Shall the similia in one, or the similia in several be accepted; shall the similia be the fantastic aberration, or the physiological counterpart? So we seek out the possible law of combination, and adapt our Specific similia to the Pathological Individuality.

With all progress, and every improvement, there comes the wail of dissatisfaction and reproach. These are avoiders of honest toil, scalers of Heaven's walls without faith or purity, who seek by a broader road the mysteries of life; indolent ones, who, while they neither toil nor spin, yet affect the gorgeous array of Solomon. But what is progress but a lessening of human toil! If it gives increased certainty of result, all the better. From the beginning, every improvement diminished somebody's work; made some hours of toil superfluous, so that this reproach becomes a praise.

That some obscurity should overshadow the pathway that leads from disease out into the highway of health, seems inevitable. To reduce this obscurity to its minimum, should be the tireless aim of scientific effort. Should there be but one dim path, we should seek to render it plainer, less devious, and less obstructed. Should there be many, we will reverently uncover our heads, and be thankful. Multitudes having gone along in the simple, open path of Specific medicine, have been led to the Elysium of health, and with gratitude acknowledge the blessing. It is to afford additional light to the thousands yet in the path, that these pages are written. Additional observation and experience will doubtless suggest improvements, giving simplicity to the direction, and certainty to the result, yet such as it is, it is offered in confidence that it will afford substantial aid to thousands.

F. HUMPHREYS, M. D.

22 West 39th Street,
*New York, April,* 1872.

# INTRODUCTION.

# Life---Health---Disease.

## LIFE.

Medicine can only have to do with living bodies. So soon as the vital principle has departed, it only remains that the body be cast off, or returned by dissolution, to its original elements.

All living bodies exist by virtue of their inherent vital principle, through which they are enabled to appropriate for their growth, development and sustentation, the elements necessary for that purpose. Through this vital principle they take up, and combine in new relations and forms, and for new offices or uses, the surrounding particles in earth, water, air, light and heat, all that may be necessary for their growth, development, and perfection. Thus all nature is constantly undergoing change, by virtue of the vital principle appropriate to each living body. With each vital principle there is the power of forming itself after its like, and of necessity, of appropriating those particles from surrounding nature which are requisite for this purpose.

Thus the acorn has in itself a germinal life, by virtue of which it first appropriates the nutriment of the nut for the development of its first shoot and rudimentary leaves, and then throwing down its spongioles or roots, begins to take up from earth and absorb from air, light and moisture the elements, from which, in a century, the sturdy monarch of the forest is produced. Every particle of all that immense tree, from rootlet to leaf, and from the outer bark to the core, the form and color, taste and odor of every leaf and twig, of every branch and bud, is determined by virtue of this inherent vital energy, which has appropriated the particles necessary for that purpose. And while it has the power to select and appropriate for its growth and sustentation what is necessary for that purpose, it has also within it certain limits of the power of rejecting that which is unsuitable or injurious. By virtue of this principle an oak is always an oak, a cherry, a parsnip or potato, is only a cherry, parsnip or potato.

If circumstances are favorable, if the plant or germ is not weak in its original inception, from parental defect, or in its germinal existence, and if surrounded by favoring circumstances in earth, air, light or heat, we may expect the full and entire development of the plant or tree, according to its order. But should these conditions be wanting, there will be variations in growth, development, or perfection, according to the degree in which the wanting substance is necessary, which may vary from the slightest deviation, down through all stages of morbid or stunted growth and imperfection, to the entire cessation of life and the dissolution of the plant itself. The entire habit of a tree may even be changed by a systematic perversion of the laws of its life.

What is true in regard to vegetable life, growth and development, holds in perhaps a higher sense in regard to animal life. In the former, vitality simply appropriates that within its reach and needful for its sustentation, unmoved by any influence higher than the Chemico-vital laws of its existence. But in animal life all these functions become complicated or more or less influenced by the psychological or mental organization of the individual. The sensible organization of man begins with a simple cyst, too small the unassisted eye to detect. This cyst, so diminutive and formless, without body or parts, is endowed with wonderful vital powers, by virtue of which it draws from the blood of the mother all that is necessary for the perfection of its embryo or fœtal life, until this form of existence, having been perfected, it is ushered into the world. Thence forward a new mode of life takes place. Through food and drink, light and air, heat and moisture, every thing required for the growth, development and sustenance of the body, is appropriated to its proper office and use, until, in this manner, man, the highest development of animal life, becomes a microcosm, having in his own body, certainly all the more common, and probably every primary element in existence. Thus we have carbon and oxygen, nitrogen and hydrogen, sulphur and iron, phosphorus and lime, ammonia and albumen, silica and silver, and even gold and arsenic. It is not probable that there is a single essential element or primate in nature that is not in a more or less perfected condition found in the body of man. The bones are mostly phosphate and carbonate of lime. Sulphur prevails largely in the skin, hair and nails, and phosphorus in the brain, silica forms the enamel of the teeth and the white of the eye, and through all this wonderful structure, each element plays its essential part, and not only sustains that part, but serves to maintain the integrity of the whole. It is not to be supposed that these chemical elements exist within us in their gross or crude forms. In some cases they exist in considerable quantities, but always progressed, or in a degree of refinement far beyond what is observed in their usual or gross forms, and in many cases they exist in forms so minute, and proportions so diminutive as only to be detected by the most delicate tests which science has been able to invent. Nay, the condition in which they often exist is, if possible, infinitely more refined or attenuated than the most extended Homeopathic potence of the same element. Each of these particles is appropriated or eliminated from the material taken, and each is progressed or perfected, and then placed in its proper organ, tissue or part, giving form, color, strength or other quality to the part by virtue solely of this vital principle, first called into action in the original germ. Whenever it is found that the elementary particles, necessary for the perfection of a particular tissue, part or organ, are wanting, not having been either supplied at all, or insufficiently, or in improper condition, or when the organism has failed to eliminate them from the elements presented, defect and disease must be the result, and this will be grave or trifling, in proportion as the wanting elements are essential to the integrity of the part or whole. Not merely are new particles taken up and appropriated to the growth and maintenance of each organ or tissue, but through the entire body the process of renovation is constantly going on; old, effete and worthless particles are being removed and cast off, while new and fresh ones are constantly being deposited. What we observe of the growth of the hair and nails is but an exhibition of what is going on in every part of the system. The bones change slowly, while the soft parts fill up or shrink away, sometimes in a few hours, but each is constantly undergoing changes up to the final hour of dissolution. Thus the entire body is a vast Chemico-vital laboratory, constantly taking up new elements and forming new combinations, while eliminating and dissolving and casting off old and effete particles.

All that has been observed thus far in regard to the growth and sustentation of man has reference to his unconscious existence. The heart beats, the blood is changed, the food is digested and bile secreted, whether we wake or sleep, or will or nill. Fortunately these vital functions are not placed under the control of our conscious volition. Thus far we have considered the body only with reference to its vital powers and physical organization, leaving out of view the higher plane of our existence, the psychological or mental. But with sentient beings there is not merely a vegetative or animal life, but a higher plane of spiritual life, including our entire conscious existence, all that thinks and reflects, wills and remembers, hopes and fears, and which constitutes our true self, including all our spiritual or psychological plane of existence, and to the sustentation of which in this life or form of existence, tne entire body is but the organ or temple. This spiritual or psychological existence is so intimately connected with the material form through which it manifests itself, that the growth and development of the one and the happiness and peace of the other are inseparable, and the dissolution of the one is the cessation of the visible manifestation of the other. Neither the body nor its parts can suffer or undergo destructive change in any degree without the manifestation of uneasiness, pain or suffering in the spiritual plane of its existence; and the slightest psychological changes produce corresponding changes in the body. All our passions, our hopes or fears, our joys and sorrows are reflected upon the physical organism with which we are connected. A pleasant surprise causes the blood to mantle the cheek with blushes, while fear not merely blanches the cheek and sends the blood to the vitals, but sometimes whitens the hair in a night. Thinking brings the blood to the brain, joy causes the heart to palpitate, grief or chagrin arrests the digestion, while despondency or fear always tends to typhus. Habits of living, thought or reflection, eventually stamp themselves upon the organism, so that the lines of the face eventually show the settled habit of thought. The "goodness of the hearth causeth the face to shine." The benevolent man carries his heart in his countenance, while envy or hate, avarice or treachery eventually wear themselves into furrows in the face. Thus every passion or emotion of our sentient life has its corresponding influence upon our vegetative existence, while in turn the perfection of our animal life has much, nay, almost everything to do with the peace and happiness of our higher existence. Thousands of children are considered cross and fretful, simply because they are ill, and multitudes of men are sour, morose and disagreeable from indigestion, and not a few become even felons and outlaws from a faulty or ill-balanced material organization.

While vitality has the power of appropriating from the elements presented all that may be necessary for the development and sustenance of the body, it has also a power of discrimination and of rejection within certain limits of that which is hurtful or inimical to its integrity or existence. In this sense life has been termed a force of resistance. No sooner are inimical or hurtful substances taken into the system, than the vital powers set up a process tending to their expulsion. In some cases the opposition is so forcible and sudden as to call up the most extraordinary manifestations, while in others it seems necessary that a longer and more tedious series of means should be adapted for the same end. The first is most clearly seen in the action of the system against those substances which are so prejudicial, as to have obtained the name of poisons. In such cases the most revulsive efforts are manifested and the system seeks by vomiting, purging, fever, sweating, or other exciting efforts, to rid itself of substances injurious or inimical to its peace and integrity. So when articles improper in quantity or quality have been taken, an action is set up, more or less violent or determined, with a view of throwing off the offending substance. Such action, though it has in view and tends to re-establish the equilibrium of the system, is, nevertheless, morbid and is properly termed disease. In some cases the offending matter is at once thrown off and the system promptly rights itself, while in others it is only after a long course of depression, violent febrile action and prostration, that the system finally rallies, or it may be exhausted and sink under its excessive efforts. Substances appropriate for our growth and sustentation in proper quantities, become prejudicial and life inimical if taken when deteriorated in quality or excessive in quantity. Some articles of food can only be taken with impunity in small quantities, while others may be taken safely in any amount and at almost any time. Nor can all persons, even when in good health, take the same articles or quantities, with equal satisfaction or impunity, nay, there are some to whom eggs are as poisonous as can well be described, while to others, onions or lobster, or even roses or honey are substances of their constant fear or dread; and these articles, usually so innocent or harmless to others, act upon them with the violence of poisons, inflicting not only great suffering, but serious and even lasting sickness. The reason would seem to be that vitality in these various cases, has no need in her economy of these peculiar elements or combinations of them that are presented in these examples, and hence revolts against them as against other noxia or poisons.

Not merely these antipathies, but also the longings so common among certain persons, may be referred to the same instinctive source. It is said that animals instinctively seek and eat plants or substances known to be beneficial for their particular diseases. Cattle afflicted with what is termed bone disease—a peculiar softening of the bones—

seek and gnaw with avidity, bones which contain phosphate of lime, the particular element wanting in their system. Deer, it is said, bury their horns as they fall off in the spring, and again resort to them from time to time, and by devcuring them, refurnish the material for the immense and rapid growth of the new antlers. The longing for water, and cooling, acidulated drinks in fevers, is as natural as it is during the heat of summer, arising in either case from the excessive evaporation in the form of sweat or insensible perspiration, resulting in the rapid exhaustion of moisture from the blood and soft parts, and hence vitality calling in these longings for the needed supply. The desire of children or girls of a certain age for chalk, clay, slate or similar substances may doubtless be referred to some chemical want of the system, of which this longing is the expression. It will be observed that these longings mostly occur during some particular state or condition of the system, when it is about to establish some change or evolution, and hence, some extraordinary expenditure is required. Hence, females when about to establish the menstruation or during the process of maturity, when all the elements for a new organization are to be eliminated, are most subject to them. In some organizations there may be primary deficiencies which are never fully supplied, and the manifestation of longings or eccentricities of appetite or want, are rarely or never absent.

We have seen that vitality has the power of selecting and appropriating whatever is necessary to perfect itself after its own material and form, and has also a wonderful power of overcoming obstacles and adapting itself to circumstances.

True, the perfection of the organism must arise from the ample and appropriate nature of the material afforded, yet a modified and seemingly healthy condition is often found under very adverse circumstances. An oak may be systematically dwarfed to a yard in height, and yet manifest its complete identity. So Animal Life is found in a thousand instances, thriving and striving against influences the most injurious or inimical. The potato grows in the dark cellar, even though the light can give no color to its vine, and eyeless fish swim in the waters of the Mammoth Cave. Whole races of men live almost exclusively upon rice and fruits, while others live as exclusively upon the fat of the whale or seal. The secretion of the salivary glands is supposed to be quite beneficial to health, but millions, by the systematic use of tobacco, deprive themselves of saliva. Good air, cleanliness and wholesome food are considered indispensable to health, yet the thousands of children playing in the gutters of our large cities, reeking with foul odors and covered with dirt, and yet comparatively tough and hearty,show that vitality can yet maintain its integrity, even against these malign influences; nay, there are those who habitually take ardent spirits, tobacco, opium, and even arsenic for years, or even half a life time, and yet poor depressed vitality succeeds in affording them a sort of quasi health, notwithstanding. That men live in apparent health, even under these malign influences, proves, not that the influences themselves are uninjurious or harmless, but that vitality, at least for a time possesses a power of self-sustentation, which over-rides their destructive tendencies.

Similar to this is the faculty possessed by the organism

and its several parts of adaptacion to circumstances, in order to accomplish what may be required of it. The limits of human endurance or accomplishment are almost beyond comprehension, and things are every day done which at first sight seem impossible. So soon as a demand is made upon the system or an organ, vitality sets in operation the means to accomplish that result. If the resources are properly husbanded and the end perseveringly sought, vitality will sooner or later, more or less perfectly, according to the circumstances, respond to that requirement. The eye of the watch-maker becomes wonderfully acute in the perception of small objects, while that of the pilot discovers objects at distances impossible to others. The touch of the blind enables him to read, while the eye of the deaf detects the words of another from the motion of the lips.

Sometimes an organ or faculty becomes so changed from education or habit, as to become perverted, or an entire new faculty may be called into existence. The miller awakes when the mill stops, and the night watchman sleeps best in the day time. Those who have long followed the proving of drugs upon themselves, and hence have long and constant occasion to analyze their own sensations and functions, find an entirely new faculty called into existence, of which before they had been ignorant. In the effort of vitality to adapt itself to circumstances, to exist even if not according to its original type, new forms or modifications are constantly manifested. The following out of these new forms under the same or similar circumstances, give rise to permanently new varieties. Thus domestic animals or fowls exhibit almost every variety of color or even shape, while the wild are unvarying in color and form. The wild goose or pigeon are always the same, while domestic ones, limited in their supplies, are subjected to arbitrary crossings, exhibit great variety of form and color. Deviations in the flowering of plants or the production of fruit or grain are referrible originally to the same source. True, all nature tends to perfection. But in order to perfection there must be varieties, that the most beneficial of these be propagated while the imperfect are permitted to perish.

---

## HEALTH.

When the influence of vitality is undisturbed, and the organism is supplied with its necessary pabulum or nourishment, health is the result. In this condition the play of the vital forces through the organism and the ministrations of the organism in return, to the higher behest of our being are in harmony, the performance of every function and indeed every action is attended with pleasurable sensations, nay, there is a happiness in mere existence. The ceaseless twitter or song of the birds, the gambol of fishes or the humming or dancing of insects in the sun, all betray the happiness realized in mere healthy existence. The digestion of the food, the circulation of the blood or the thousand sensations going on in every portion of our complex organism, are all sources of enjoyment, while the attainment of knowledge, the performance of benevolent actions, or of the higher offices of our being, are attended with the highest sense of enjoyment to the individual. The sense of this enjoyment in health calls into exercise the highest activities of our being, and it is only when they are over taxed, or illy adjusted by ill health, or perverted, that their performance ceases to afford gratification. To this gratification we owe the ceaseless energy that illuminates the higher achievements of our race.

Modified health is not incompatible with deviations in form or even mutilation or loss of parts. Doubtless the highest health is found connected with the most perfect type and symmetrical form, but nature, in the case of deviations or deformities, or even mutilations, adapts herself to circumstances and still maintains her integrity, as far as the conditions will admit. The leg of the dancer or the arm of the smith, increased to twice their natural size, from long continued exercise, cannot be considered unhealthy, nor yet the diminished muscle of the professional man, whose non use has failed to call out its full development. In the law of our being, to adapt each part to its requirements, we notice constant deviations from what might be considered the most complete order or symmetry, so that breeds of animals or races of men assume forms or changes of structure or proportion that are very striking. In the progress of the human race there is an age of muscle, and then an age of brains, and vitality adapting each to its want and training, fashions its race accordingly. That undoubtedly is most nearly perfect which is best adapted to its use. The heart of one man may be twice the size of that of another and yet be perfectly healthy, having a corresponding arterial and nervous system, while in some delicate individuals it may be very small, with a pulse like that of a bird, yet both are healthy. One person has an exceedingly delicate nervous organization, while another has so little nervous development as to be almost insensible to pain or even to pleasure. One feels exquisitely every passing emotion or passion, while to another they scarcely exist. Yet none of these can properly be called deviations from the standard of health. Each may be healthy according to its standard.

The inherent vitality of the individual has much to do with his power of self-sustentation, and hence of preserving health. We inherit from our parents, not merely the type and form, the complexion and habits of body, the temperament and tendencies of the organism, but also about so many years of existence. Other things being equal, the son will live about as many years as did his father, and the daughter as her mother. Temperance and observance of the laws of life will add a few years to the thread, or evil habits and dissipation will shorten it somewhat, but in the average a man may expect to live about the age of his father, while all are of course liable to be cut off by accidents or acute diseases. With some the hold on life is much stronger than in others, and they will not only live longer but withstand influences to which others speedily succumb. A rat often outlives the most terrible mutilations, while a rabbit may be killed by the slightest blow. Some persons outlive the most terrible ravages of disease, while others die before they are supposed to be in danger. Some persons are so constituted that every passing influence affects them. They have all the disease incident to childhood, and during adult life every passing influence, dysentery, influenza, cholera, diphtheria or other epidemic, finds an arena in their system, while there are others whose vitality rides safely and without injury through all such malign influences. Nay, there are those who seem proof against even small-pox, syphilis or yellow fever. It would seem that vitality in these cases holds the organism so perfectly under its control as to render it proof against influences which are so frequently fatal to others.

As health is the harmonious action and balance of the vital force and the various functions of the organism, it follows that the more complex or delicate the structure or organism, the more liable it becomes to fall into disorder or disease. Every additional element that enters into the organization, is an additional influence whose action must be in union with every part and with the whole in order to its healthy or harmonious action. Vegetable life may only suffer from the quality or quantity of the material which makes up the structure. Animal life may still further suffer from the sentient system which forms a part of its organism, while in intelligent beings the whole is still further complicated by that immense sway of psychological phenomena, that thinking and willing, hoping and fearing, whose ebb and flow is more or less reflected upon every plane of the being below it. Hence, the more refined, delicate and sensitive the organism becomes, the more nicely and delicately are its balances adjusted, the more exquisite are its perceptions and enjoyments, the keener is grief or depressions and the more liable to become ill-adjusted and to fall into disorder. Time was in the history of the race when diseases were very few and proportionately fatal, but with the progress and development of man they have increased a hundred fold, because there are a hundred more influences in play, all of which must be in harmony in order to the perfect result. This is seen in the difference between wild and domestic animals. Wild birds or animals are subject to few or no diseases, and not until after many generations of domestication do they become subject to them, while the thorough-bred horse or dog must be treated as tenderly as a child. The Indian has but few diseases, and those of an acute character and generally fatal, while the fully cultured and developed man or woman is the subject of almost numberless morbid influences.

---

## DISEASE.

When the organism or any of its parts falls into disordered action, it is said to be *diseased*. The first manifestations of disease are usually upon the highest planes of the organism. Not until after these have been invaded and their action modified by the morbid process, does it descend to the lower or more material planes of the organism. Thus it is first the psychological or moral, then the sensational, then the functional, and last of all the material plane of our being that is invaded. The first perceptions of diseased action are sensation of depression, melancholy or misanthropy, or they may assume a more violent or positive form of sadness, ill humor or mental alienation in various forms or degrees. In some instances the morbid process does not ultimate itself in lower planes, but expends its force in the first arena of its action, and the result may be insanity or hypochondria, or some similar form of permanent mental alienation. But in the usual course the next plane of the organism, the sensational is invaded, and there are then manifestations of pain, uneasiness, aching or weariness. Some morbid conditions, such as neuralgia, are characterized almost exclusively by these manifestations. Next, the functions of the body become disordered, the appetite fails, taste becomes impaired, tongue coated, secretions obstructed, and some or all of the functions of the body are perverted, or more or less impaired or arrested. In some cases the principal sphere of the morbid process is the perversion of a function, as in case of diarrhœa or diabetes. Lastly, we come to alterations of structure—the localization of disease upon the material plane. Here we may have redness, swelling and heat, as in inflammations, or, lesions of parts, as in ulcers, or changes in the structure of the part or even its ultimate molecules, as in case of cancer or scirrhus. In particular instances the invasion of the organism may be so sudden that its successive steps or stages may not be marked, and the entire system may seem to be affected at once, or some of its planes may seem to have been glided over and scarcely assailed, or in so slight a manner as to have been unnoticed, or the morbid manifestation may be so positive or decided in some one particular field as to give the impression that that is the only plane of the morbid process. Yet before any of these changes of structure could have occurred it is evident there must have been also changes in the vital being, to which only by slow degrees the change of structure was eventually made to correspond.

The recuperative or healthward manifestations of the system proceed in the same order. The first perception of relief is in the moral sphere—the patient feels more cheerful, less depression gloom or irritability, then relief from pain and uneasiness, sleep and countenance more natural; then, the functions are improved, circulation, taste, appetite, and secretions more regular and normal, and finally the conditions of structure, if there has been organic lesions, gradually assume a more natural and healthy character. Often during the height of a malady a single appropriate dose of the required remedy is given, and the patient at once becomes more calm and quiet, and sleep comes on, giving most indubitable evidence to the appreciating mind that vitality has been relieved and a healthward process established. The curative process commences in the highest sphere and from thence descends to the lower and more material plane.

In case of wounds, injuries, or lesions of parts, the first injury may be in the material structure, yet the perceptions of the morbid process and the curative manifestations of the system are first indicated in the higher and more immaterial planes of the organism. In some instances a morbid process may be so remote from the seat of life, and so little effect its normal functions, as to call but very slightly into play its sympathetic action, and such cases have been erroneously termed local diseases, such as indolent ulcers, tumors, or adventitious growths.

The genesis of disease presents some interesting considerations. Unquestionably the early progenitors of the race were not subject to all the diseases which are now common. The advent of many are well known. When an individual or community has for a long period violated the laws of life or health, the violation seems to ultimate itself in the form of a particular corresponding malady or disease, which having once ultimated itself in that particular form, assumes a type, and hence, constantly tends to reproduce itself in new subjects. Thus the cholera was first known during the early part of the present century. Among the crowded and ill-fed masses of India, exposed to pestilential miasm from sluggish rivers, among swamps and rice fields, there was developed a peculiar form of disease, which first rioted in its own home, sweeping off hundreds of thousands of the wretched inhabitants; until after a few years, it stretched out first along the water courses and great lines of travel, until at length it overleaped all sanitary cordons, visited in turn all the great cities of Europe and America, and finally became known as the cholera in almost every part of the habitable globe. So the plague, doubtless engendered by the peculiar habits and endemic influences of the Levant at times stretches out its malignant folds and involves London, Paris and other distant and usually exempt cities. The yellow fever is usually confined to the low miasmatic coasts of the Southern portion of this country and similar tropical regions, but at times it has been known to travel inland and visit places hundreds of miles beyond its original locality. Syphilis was unknown until about the year of 1495, when it first appeared at Naples, and has since extended to every part of the habitable world. The advent of many diseases of modern date are well known and easily marked. In the course of many years the character and peculiarities of a disease may become changed or modified, or it may entirely disappear, while other diseases or new manifestations may take their place. New diseases or new forms of familiar ones are constantly coming forward, and will be likely to do so as long as the habits of the race and surrounding influences are subjects of corresponding changes.

It is not strange that diseases run in similar channels, or that a type constantly tends to reproduce itself. The human organization being always mainly the same, a morbid influence acting upon it elicits mainly the same response or symptoms. The shadings may be varied by the peculiarities of the subject and potency of the exciting cause, but the essential features will be similar. In some cases the morbid influence is so positive that it always elicits the same symptoms only varied in their degree or intensity, and these have obtained the name of diseases of fixed character. Small-pox and measles have far less variety than scarlet fever, owing doubtless to the varying degree of intensity in the morbid cause. All epidemics are observed to have their rise, acme and declination, as well as to vary in their character and degree of intensity from year to year.

From these considerations it will be seen that disease is not to be considered as a material, something which has got into the system and hence is to be expelled from it, but as primarily *a deviation from the normal standard in the play of the immaterial vital forces* that govern and control the material organism. These deviations, which we term disease, arise in a large majority of cases from causes which are as immaterial as the vital being itself. In some cases the causes may indeed be material—poisons, bad food, excesses, wounds, etc., which, acting through the material organism upon the immaterial forces within it, derange the play of the entire organism; but often they are of the most immaterial character. The cholera swept off its thousands and even decimated the population of some large cities and communities, yet that was no rational solution for its presence found in air, earth or water, or even yet in the surrounding electrical conditions of the atmosphere. Nor has the presence of scarlet fever, diphtheria, or typhus been detected in any material form aside from their manifestations. The most delicate tests applied to an atmosphere reeking with fever and ague, yellow fever or small-pox, fail to detect a difference between them and that of the most salubrious mountain region. Yet an atmosphere apparently innocuous may be so charged with malaria or contagion as to destroy a large proportion of all susceptible persons who come within its reach. In inflammation, fever, rheumatism, a mere check of perspiration or sudden exposure, gives rise to all the phenomena of the disease, without the possibility of any material cause having contributed to the disorder. When changes in the structure of the part have occurred, such changes are not to be considered the cause of disease but the result or consequence of morbid action. Usually quite a period of time is required, and a series of immaterial changes or evolutions of the organism are necessary before any material alteration of structure can occur. This is very manifest in cases of cancer, tumor, or similar lesions of structure.

## HOW MEDICINES CURE.

All crude medicines are in their nature poisons or health-destroying agencies. By virtue of their ability to disturb health, they have, under certain circumstances, the power to restore it. But it is not necessary, in order to restore health, that medicines be used in quantities sufficient to disturb or destroy it. Homeopathy has fortunately shown the world how medicine can be so used as to restore, without the possibility of injuring, and how to develop the curative powers of medicine, while their poisonous properties are destroyed.

It has been common to use emetics, cathartics, sudorifics or expectorants, with a view of promoting the excretions of the body, that thereby disease might be expelled and health recovered; and it is not doubted that after the operation of a brisk cathartic or emetic, the patient has frequently been restored. But as during the operation of the medicine it may in many cases be shown that every grain of the drug administered, except an immaterial Homeopathic portion, has been ejected from the system, it becomes a question whether the large quantity which has been thrown off or the immaterial small quantity (Homeopathic) which remained, has been the curative agent. Surely the mechanical effort of vomiting or purging has no more curative action than the wiping of one's nose has in curing the catarrh, and the fact that Homeopaths do cure with the small portion, confirms the impression that all the large dose and revulsive operation was at least misapplied. In very few cases will these mechanical manipulations cure disease.

No fact is better settled than that Homeopathic medicines cure. The method of their operation has been variously explained. Even should it not be susceptible of explanation at all, or upon any generally accepted principle or hypothesis, yet this would not invalidate the fact of such cures; or should any of the usual explanations prove to be incorrect, yet the fact still stands, only the supposed rationale has proved fallacious. Homeopathic cures, if not all cures by medicine, seem to be upon the principle of SUBSTITUTION. To substitute a similar, medicinal action for a morbid one, is to extinguish disease. In some cases this may be easy, in others difficult, or again impossible, as every art of necessity has its limits. This cure by substitution or Homeopathy is not new, the truth flashed from the immortal poet when he sung—

> " Tut man, one fire burns out another's burning,
> Turn giddy, and be helped by backward turning,
> Take some new infection to thine eye,
> And the rank poison of the old will die."

Applying snow to the frost-bitten parts, and heating applications to burns, are familiar examples. But the cure of syphilitic diseases by mercurials, or of fever and ague by quinine, or sore throat by cayenne pepper, are as truly Homeopathic as the former, and all truly specific or curative medicines will be found to range themselves under this principle of action—the Homeopathic.

All prevention of disease is upon this (Homeopathic) principle. Vaccinnation, with the kine-pock, prevents the small-pox, because the mode of action and the essential phenomenon of the two diseases are similar in the course they run, the symptoms they produce, the local swelling and scar they leave behind; and being thus similar the one acts as a substitute for the other. The kine-pock as truly protecting the system as does the small-pox itself from a second attack. Minute doses of quinine prevent fever and ague and other malarious fevers, and belladonna prevents scarlet fever upon the same principle.

In Homeopathy, we first ascertain by proving or trials of medicines upon the healthy, the organs or tissues upon which such drugs act, by observing the symptoms or disturbances in the system which they produce. Having thus, by repeated trials, learned the affinities of every medicine, we are enabled to apply them with great certainty in disease. Because, if a disease or morbid condition produces certain symptoms, and a medicine produces the same or similar symptoms, it is certain it must do so by acting upon the same organs and tissues, and in the same manner, and thus to give the same, we substitute, if it is possible, the one *medicinal* for the other *morbid* action, and thus substituting, cure it. And here our use of minute doses finds explanation. Few diseases produce the symptoms of large material doses, or if they did, such large doses assault the system so violently, as to call up a revulsive action, which convulses, torments and poisons, while it does not cure. But Homeopathic doses acting upon a higher plane of the organism, that upon which disease begins, gradually and sometimes immediately substitute their action for that of disease, and thus modify, soften and extinguish it. The dose or amount of medicine given must be in harmony with the condition of the vital forces when it is given. It often happens that a very minute dose will act curatively, when a larger one will not so act at all, and it is a very gross but common error to suppose that if a little medicine will do some good, a larger quantity will do more good. It is often quite the contrary.

As medicines have special affinities for different organs or tissues, as for instance, belladonna for the eye and brain, mercury for the glands and sulphur for the skin, etc.; the rationale of this action must be the affinity of the medicine for homogeneous particles of the same element in the human system. As the human body is a microcosm, having in itself the known primary elements, it follows that every one of these elements or its combinations may become a medicine, and by its influence serve to modify and control the action of the organism through its influence upon homogeneous particles of the same element in the human system. These elements, as they exist in the human body are in a condition infinitely more refined and progressed than the condition in which they are found elsewhere. Hence it is that in order to act curatively, as medicines, and in the most speedy and efficient manner, they must be reduced, triturated, refined and attenuated so as at least to approximate to the condition in which they exist in the human body. Thus refined, attenuated and progressed they are no longer poisons or health-disturbing agents, but on the contrary are life-sustainers, vital pabulums, in every way conserving and sustaining the health and vigor of the body, not only curing disease when rightly applied, but protecting and preventing disease and decay. In this condition the poisonous properties of medicines are destroyed and their curative or conservative ones are developed. And therein we have an answer to that stale and crude fallacy urged by the thoughtless, that because a child might eat a bottle full of Homeopathic medicine and not be poisoned, hence, such medicine could have no power to cure the sick. Specific Homeopathy especially recognizes this fundamental principle — that medicines act curatively through their affinities with homogeneous particles of the same elements in the system. Hence, in the formation of every specific, we seek, not merely to give a simple, which may act in a certain direction or upon a certain organ or tissue, but to unite in a specific medicine, elements, which having the same direction or symptoms, yet act upon fundamentally different elements or tissue in the body. This is done by combining medicines of widely different constituent principles or elements, and while each of these is Homeopathic to the disease, they sustain the system differently by acting upon different organs, tissues, nerve centres, or organic elements. Thus, while one may serve as pabulum for the blood, another may perform the same office for the bones, while a third may directly act upon the nervous system, and all may conduce to a general result. Vegetable poisons, animal poisons, chemicals, minerals and metals, as classes, each act differently upon the human system, and each perform offices which can not well be performed by others, and the great advantage of Specific Homeopathy is that specifics are formed that unite in one Homeopathic preparation the virtues of these several classes of medicines. Results are by this means attained, not only in the simplicity of the application, but also in the certainty and value of the results, especially in the cure of obstinate and long-standing diseases, which are not realized by any other method.

Numerous morbid conditions arise from the deprivation of some element essential to the integrity of the system—as the want of iron in the blood, or of phosphate and carbonate of lime in the bones. These substances administered, not in crude, but in refined or Homeopathic forms, are found to act like enchantment in supplying the wanting substance, not so much perhaps in giving the quantity required as by setting in action the inchoate particles of the same elements already present. When it is remembered that these elementary particles, as they exist in our blood, our organs, our tissues and bones are usually in particles, so exceedingly minute and refined, as at times only to be detected by the most delicate tests which chemistry has discovered, it will be comprehended that in order to act affinitively upon such particles, the element given as a medicine must be attenuated or reduced to a similar condition, or one approximating it. True, the mortar and pestle, with sugar of milk, will never reduce sulphur to the condition of that which plays so essential a part in the human system, even though the pestle be held or the bottle shaken by a benevolent and healthy hand. But this mode of preparation is the nearest to perfection and has attained the highest results yet known in the experience of man. And it may be also admitted that by this mode of preparation there is imparted to the medicine, not merely a fineness in its form, but also some portion of the vital electricity or power of the individual performing the manipulation or making the medicine. As the condition of an electrical current is modified in passing from the machine through the organism of another individual to the patient, so the direct Homeopathic manipulation of a medicine by a healthy and well-disposed person, is not without its influences in sustaining and restoring the sick.

In the permanent restoration of the sick, especially in long standing or chronic diseases, time is required. Often such diseases are of many years standing, and have by degrees involved every plane of the organism, producing disturbances of function and sensation, and even changes in the structure or tissues of the body itself. When it is realized that all these must be changed, renovated or even renewed by efforts of the immaterial vital forces, assisted by the kindly influence of medicine appropriate in quality, quantity, form and repetition, and sustained by appropriate nutrition, it will be seen that health, under such circumstances, can not be the work of a day or week; and the patient should be content even if months or years are required for permanent and entire recovery. In some marvelous cases the power of disease may be broken at once, and the change produced be so great that the patient believes himself well. In almost all cases where a cure is possible, the appropriate medicine produces an improvement at once, or in a very few days, but in most cases experience has abundantly shown that time, repeated doses, and a persistent use of appropriate medicine, are required for the cure of serious and long-standing diseases.

In many instances the medicinal influence is soon extinguished or lost, so that repeated doses are required for a cure, while in others, a single dose, permitted to expend its action undisturbed, has produced the most important changes and even annihilated a long-standing and obstinate disease. Some diseases run their course rapidly, and their cure may be as rapidly effected, while others are months and even years working out a morbid process, and often require a similar range of time for their permanent annihilation and cure.

## CAUSES OF DISEASE.

### HEREDITARY TRANSMISSION.

It is not unfrequently observed that a family are all subject to some peculiar disease or morbid condition, and that father and son, mother and daughter, by turn, are subject to the same disease, or that a certain disease runs in particular families. Sometimes nearly a whole family die in the course of a few years from consumption, or that sons are afflicted with gout, scrofula, salt rheum or rheumatism, as their father was before them, or that daughters inherit cancer from mothers or grandmothers. The impression hence generally prevails that these diseases are inherited. The fact of disease frequently appearing under such circumstances is undisputed. However difficult it may be to conceive how the vital principle, in forming for itself a body, shall, from some inherent defect or weakness, form it of materials, which at a certain period of life are subject to disease or dissolution in a certain form, it is quite certain that as each parent imparts to its offspring its own type and peculiarities, its tendency to be lean or corpulent, large or small, delicate or stout, so with this bodily organization there is a tendency to assume or take on diseased action in a certain form. A family—father and sons—may all have a large body and short neck, and large arterial system, and hence, at certain periods of life be very liable to apoplexy. So in a peculiar conformation or habit of body there will be a strong tendency to tuberculous deposits, and hence, consumption. We do not, perhaps, so much inherit a disease as we do a peculiar make or habit of body and temperament, which is very liable to assume a particular form of disease.

It is not usually difficult to arrest such tendencies in the bud, by the appropriate use of Homeopathic medicines, and they only require to be understood and guarded against by proper habits and medication, in order to ward off danger from such sources. The medicines and measures of prevention against such disease will be indicated in their appropriate sections.

## MIASMS.

Often, over extensive sections of country, and sometimes successively over vast regions, people are afflicted with some peculiar form of disease, such as influenza, cholera, scarlet fever, etc. The influence which causes such diseases is unknown. It is observed to have its beginning, reach a certain degree of intensity,and then to decline. During its presence all susceptible persons are more or less afflicted by it, yet only a portion of the entire population are attacked with the disease. Other diseases, during its continuance, are variously modified and made to wear the livery of the prevailing epidemic. All patients will not have the same symptoms, but all will have the more important or peculiar ones, showing the unity of the miasmatic influence. While all are doubtless within its influence, wherever it extends, yet, beyond question, the miasm or disease-producing agency is more intense in the immediate vicinity of those who have the disease, and to this extent it may be considered contagious. A susceptible person coming into the immediate presence of those who are laboring under the disease, is doubtless more exposed than elsewhere, as the morbid influence is there more intense. Fear, or an apprehensive state of mind, renders the person more susceptible than otherwise, while a calm, quiet and determined state of mind is not without its influence as a protective, vitality being thus placed in the best possible position to resist the invasion.

Not unfrequently the epidemic influence seems to change its mode of manifestation, and one disease is found to follow another. Thus the cholera has been very commonly preceded by the influenza, the diphtheria by scarlet fever, and dysentery by intermittent fever.

## ENDEMIC CAUSES.

Diseases are frequently engendered by local or endemic influences. Thus, the neighborhood of swamps and marshes, or the drainage of ponds, almost invariably causes some grade of remittent or intermittent fevers. Persons residing in such localities are subject to these diseases, and new countries where large portions of land are being cleared and hence drained, are almost invariably subject to these fevers. So the digging of canals or extensive drains is for a time observed to be followed by similar results. When stagnant water stands in a cellar for any considerable time, the family or some of its members residing over it, will rarely escape some form of fever. There are also some diseases that seem to be peculiar to certain localities or sections of country, among which may be mentioned the Plica Polonica, or plaited hair disease of Poland, and the Goitre or Derbyshire Neck, which, in its peculiar form, is observed in certain localities, and certain forms of cretinism, observed among the deep valleys of the Alps.

## DEPRIVATION.

There are numerous cases of disease produced by the want or deprivation of some substance essential to the integrity of the system. As the organism takes up and eliminates from surrounding nature the elements essential to its perfection and integrity, it follows that if these organic elements are absent in that which is received, or found only in such form that it cannot ultimate them within itself, or, if by any fault of the organism, this ultimation or conversion cannot be accomplished, disease must of necessity follow. At times our vital being makes the most extraordinary efforts to supply these deficiencies, and may for a time succeed, but finally help must be afforded or the system must succumb. Mariners, on long voyages, or shut up in the icy regions of the North and deprived of the citric acid found in vegetables and fruit, for many months maintain a degree of health, but scurvy, ere long, makes its sad ravages, unless fruits or vegetables are obtained. Emigrants from Europe, confined for many weeks upon ship-board, pining from home-sickness, unable to eat or digest their food from sea-sickness, and exposed to uncleanliness and bad air, from over-crowded and ill-ventilated ships, suffer terribly from ship fever. Deprivation of light and air soon blanch the cheeks and give the inmates of our prisons that pale appearance, so common to old convicts.

Children not unfrequently fail to receive in the milk of the nurse all the elements necessary to the healthy formation of bone, or their systems are not in a condition to eliminate and deposit from the aliment received the proper amount of ossific matter; as a consequence the bones are formed slowly and with apparent suffering to the system, the teeth are produced slowly and irregularly, the fontanel does not close, the long bones are crooked, with large wrists and ankles, and the children are tottering, slow in learning to walk, or walk only with difficulty. The result is not only a defective osseous system, but a general innervation of the entire organism, manifested by stunted growth, imperfect development and general weakness.

In many instances there is a marked disproportion between the expenditure of the system mentally and physically, and its nourishment or sustentation. This is especially liable to occur during the years of development, or the evolutions of the system. Hence the period of puberty is so frequently critical, and if, during that period, the mental activity is over-taxed, by study or mental effort, while the sytem is insufficiently nourished, this impoverishment of the system is liable to result in the deposition of tubercles or other serious disease. Thousands die annually of consumption engendered at school, or fall an easy prey to typhus fever and other diseases, because the vital forces have been exhausted, while the organism has been insufficiently sustained by food and nourishment. The early period of nursing is frequently critical for a similar reason. The great demand made upon the system for the lacteal fluid at a period of recent exhaustion from child-bed may find the system inadequate to the supply; and hence exhaustion, successive deposition of tubercles and rapid decline is the result, unless the system be adequately sustained.

## EXHAUSTION.

Closely allied to the above condition, and similar in its consequence, is that arising from the exhaustion of the system. This may be accomplished in a variety of ways, and in this very busy and enterprising age, is often done before the victim is aware of his danger. There are multitudes of cases of paralysis, partial, or entire loss of nervous or muscular control, or both, in some portion of the body, frequently one side, which have been caused by long continuedexhausting excitement of the system. The brain ultimately becoming exhausted and its power in part destroyed, so that the muscle no longer responds to the efforts of the will. The frequency of paralysis in late years, is doubtless to be attributed to the excessive mental effort engendered but too frequently among the business community.

Excessive venery exhausts its thousands, and while it impairs the mental powers, it so far reduces the vital forces, that other causes the more readily undermine and exhaust the organism. Multitudes of mothers are enfeebled in producing and nursing their offspring. True, nature usually guards this most important of her designs with jealous care, but if there be added to the debility of pregnancy and nursing, a loss of appetite or derangement of the digestion, so that the system is insufficiently supplied with nutriment, the consequence must be weakness, deposition of tubercles and ultimate disease and dissolution unless aid be offered.

## NURSING AND CARE OF THE SICK.

Goodness of heart, a kind and obliging disposition and good sense are the indispensable elements of good nursing. Medicine, in some cases, can play but a secondary part in the cure of the sick, but good nursing, or care always plays a prominent part. The object of nursing is to place the system of the patient in the best possible condition for the beneficial action of medicine. In some cases of disease, medicine properly applied, is indispensable, while in all cases it is within the power of the patient and attendants to nullify the best efforts of medicines and physician by bad habits, bad nursing or pernicious diet or food. The physician's duty is less than half done, when he orders medicine for the patient; the larger, and possibly more important part of his duty, is to direct as to habits, diet and living of his patients, and to see that these are such as not to antagonize or nullify the effects of his medicines. All this holds with still greater force to the Homeopathic physician or nurse.

THE ROOM of a patient or invalid should be large and airy, if possible. Close, narrow, low apartments necessitate the breathing of impure or vitiated air, and if such must be used, great care must be taken in respect to ventilation. The temperature of the room should be about 70 to 75 degrees of Fahrenheit, and in dry, moderate weather the sash should be often or constantly drawn down at the top of the window for a more complete ventilation. In many instances the sash may be kept down the entire night to advantage and closed only when the patient is cold or uncomfortable from it. The patient should, however, be out of the immediate current of air. To keep the air of the room pure, everything offensive should be immediately removed from it; no slops, discharges, or broken food, or remains of meals, or dirty dishes, or soiled linen should be allowed to remain a moment. The body should be often sponged off with tepid water, under the clothes and without uncovering the person, and the body linen, damp from perspiration, should be removed daily, and fresh, dry, well aired linen supplied in its place. The hands and face of a patient may be frequently sponged with tepid or cool water, when it would be improper or inconvenient to sponge the entire body. Use no disinfectants about the room,—cologne, camphor, burnt rags, burnt vinegar and the like. They merely add another smell to the one already existing, and the compound is not an improvement. The true way is to thoroughly ventilate the room, by introducing fresh air and driving out that which is contaminated.

THE PATIENT has but one thing to do, that is to get well, and all else should be subservient to this principal object, and it is unwise, during sickness, to attempt any considerable labor or work, mental or physical. The concentration of the mind in composition, study, reading or business matters involves an expenditure of vitality, that impedes recovery and the kind influence of medicines, and inevitably prolongs sickness. The sick should not be fatigued, or over-taxed by study, company, business, or worry of any kind, but every effort should be made to render them as quiet and comfortable as possible. If visitors call, and it is often proper and cheerful for them so to do, they must not tax and annoy sick people with long stories, uninteresting subjects, or with anything that over-tasks the strength, or fatigues the patient. A short, cheerful call and pleasant face are always welcome to the sick, and a kindly interest in their case is equally so. Religious conversation is always proper, when conducted intelligently and in a proper spirit, though I hold that a sick bed is far from being a proper place for this most important of the duties of life. Books may not be wholely interdicted, but the amount and character of reading should be proportioned to the strength or mental vigor of the patient.

THE ROOM of the patient should be made cheerful as well as comfortable. Do not suffer the sick to lay all day staring at the blank wall, or at strange or unsympathising faces, but flowers, bright and fresh, pictures around the room, change of furniture, or a seat or couch at the widow, serve wonderfully to cheer and invigorate a patient. The room should be light, unless while sleeping, the sun-light being as necessary for patients almost as for plants. If you wish to have the sick sad, gloomy and desponding, keep them in dark rooms, with sombre objects, and sad unmeaning faces. Noise, bustle or loud talking are always objectionable to the sick, sometimes fearfully so to persons of weak nerves, or who are very feeble. In reading to the sick, let it be done slowly and distinctly, so as not to fatigue them to follow the reader—so of conversation. The sick room is no place for idlers, loungers, or curiosity-seekers, and all such should be summarily dispensed with. While the nurse should be all attention to the wants of the sick, yet she should avoid "fussiness" or wearying the patient with unnecessary trifles. She should go calmly and quietly about her business, doing cheerfully what is necessary to be done, while yet she does not make herself the conspicuous subject of the occasion. There is an evil which cannot be too severely condemned. It is the rage to prescribe for the sick, possessed by almost every body, under every conceivable variety of circumstances. No matter how severe the disease, or how urgent the emergency, nine out of every ten persons who call, will tell precisely what will cure the patient, and the remaining person has a doctor just on hand to do the work. Usually, the more ignorant the volunteer, the more positive they are of a cure. They who know much speak cautiously. Those who know little are very positive. Now, if a physician is in attendance, it is his business to prescribe and not that of others, and it is a very delicate piece of business, under any circumstances, to advise the friends or patient to a change of treatment or medical attendant. While a physician is in attendance, simple justice to him and the welfare of the sick, require that his directions should be followed, and his instructions obeyed. It must be a rare case indeed that justifies the interference of outsiders.

In cases of *very sick* persons, it may be advisable to call in assistance of watchers, but it should be avoided if possible. Better far have some members of the family take turns in watching, and the one in charge near at hand to be called in case of emergency. In a majority of cases, those that are called in as night watchers are stupid, sleepy, ignorant of their duties, or the wants or peculiarities of the patient, and do far more harm than good. Avoid them if possible. In most cases it is better for the mother, husband, sister, or others of the family to lie down in the room and sleep while the patient sleeps, than to have the house and patient kept awake with watchers. *The bed* and *bedding* of the sick are matters of peculiar importance. The bed should not be too high, without valance or curtains to confine the air beneath it, and it is more convenient to have it drawn out from the wall so as to get on every side of it. A simple hair mattress or sacking bottom is the best, and if feathers must be used, put one or two comfortables over the tick with the linen over them, so as to make a firm and even surface. The linen of the bed and of the patient should be changed, or at least aired and dried by the fire every day. If the same linen is to be worn again by the patient it should be dried before the fire, so as to dissipate the previous bodily exhalations with which it is saturated. It is wonderful how much ease and comfort is afforded to the sick by a light, cool bed, with thin covering, frequently arranged or made up and rendered agreeable. Often the feverish restlessness of patients is entirely removed by such little comforts.

## ACCESSORY CURATIVE MEASURES.

There are certain expedients or curative measures, which may often be resorted to by nurse or invalid, which, while they can scarcely be called parts of medical treatment, yet they are of so great value, nay, so indispensable in some cases, as to demand particular attention in a treatise on domestic medicine. Among these are especially the use of hot foot-baths and the injection-pipe.

*A hot foot-bath* may be used with benefit in all cases where we desire to equalize the circulation, diminish local congestion and even inflammation. All severe inflammations and congestions are preceded by a cold chill or rigor, during which the hands and feet become cold, the head often hot, and a shivering chill extends, often with chattering teeth and blue nails, over the whole body, lasting from a few minutes to an hour or more, and is succeeded by heat and high fever. In all similar cases the hot foot-bath soonest breaks the chill, and with it the power and often the force of the disease.

Some care and knowledge should be exercised in order to derive the greatest amount of benefit from a foot-bath. The vessel should be large and deep enough to permit the water to come well up towards the knees. The temperature of the water should be such that the feet can be kept in it without inconvenience, and another vessel of hot water should be on hand, from which, as the water becomes cooled in the bath, the hot water should be, from time to time, supplied, so that the temperature may be gradually increased during the entire bath. This should be continued from ten to twenty minutes, according to the circumstances of the case, or until the patient is relieved, the chill broken, or a general perspiration appears. Then let the feet be taken from the bath, wiped rapidly dry, with warm cloths, and wrapped up comfortably, so as to retain the heat. A foot-bath, thus administered, is one of the most efficient of domestic remedies.

Sitz-baths may be administered in a tin bath, formed for the purpose, with a back, or a very serviceable one may be made, by cutting down an ordinary barrel, with a board set in it for a back. The patient sits down in the tub, with water sufficient to come well up around the hips and over the lower abdomen, and is then covered from the neck down over the tub so as to retain the vapor, if desirable. The bath may be continued from ten to thirty minutes. In cases of congestion to the lower abdominal organs, piles and in some severe cases of dysentery, these seat-baths will be found of great value.

## INJECTIONS.

More important, however, for every family, is the use and knowledge of the injection-pipe. It is indispensable in every family. The best are of rubber, with flexible tube and a bulb, containing the pumping apparatus in the centre, from which the suction tube extends a foot or more to the reservoir or dish containing the charge. The injection is usually luke-warm water. Sometimes to a pint of water a large spoonful of molasses is added, and if a more active injection is yet required, a tablespoonful of salt may be supplied. Very generally simple tepid water is sufficient. The end of the tube should be covered with oil, cerate or lard, and then introduced by gentle manipulations into the rectum. If the object is to dislodge hardened feces, the pipe should be inserted, so as to place the water above the hardened mass. The pumping should then be continued until a pint, quart, or even double that quantity of fluid has been thrown up. Should one injection not succeed, it may be repeated after a half hour or more, until the object is obtained. In cases of obstinate constipation, a morning injection, with the use of the appropriate specific, never fails. In obstinate and violent colic, a large injection often fully relieves. In all cases of fever and threatened convulsions in children, arising from having eaten hurtful or indigestible substances—fruit, cake, raisins, oranges, etc.—the proper use of the injection-pipe, in connection with the specific medicines, will save the patient. These injections are in no instance hurtful, and are a far better expedient than the use of pills, cathartics, or even such laxatives as castor oil.

---

## FOOD.

As the growth and waste of the body must be restored and replenished by appropriate nutrition, it follows, that the best condition of body and mind will be attained by the use of that kind of nutrition best adapted to its wants. Much trouble and illness might be avoided if people only knew, and could obtain the kind of food best adapted to their special needs. Health may often be restored by the use of proper food, as sickness is often induced from the want of it. It will be impossible to specify for each individual case, but hints may be drawn by indicating the kind of food best adapted for the several classes which are mentioned. Each period of life has its most appropriate food, so has each season of the year and each habit of constitution or body, and that which is proper for one is often quite improper, and sometimes even injurious to another. The distinction is based upon chemico-vital wants of the system, at different periods of life, and under varying or varied conditions of the living body. To be more particular:

THE FOOD OF INFANTS AND YOUNG CHILDREN should contain all the elements, out of which the entire system is to be developed. There must be material for making every separate tissue of the entire man, and that in a condition to be as readily assimilated as possible. Milk from the cow meets all these conditions, having in itself all the elements required for the human body, and in their best proportions and condition. To this may be added barley, in its various forms, as of gruel, or in pap or cakes, in proportion to its age and development of teeth, the soup or flesh of beef or mutton. If the child is fat, heavy or stupid, it requires food containing more nitrates and phosphates—lean meat, oat-meal, barley cakes, bean or pea soup, &c. If too lean and thin, it may be indulged in the more stupefying carbonates, as fat meat, fine flour, butter, sugar, or puddings, pies, &c. Thus the food may be varied as the needs of the child demand.

FOOD FOR LABORING MEN should in part be adapted to the nature of their labor, and to the season or temperature. But in general, as there is a large expenditure of muscular effort, the supply should be equal to the drain. Hence, beef, mutton, a proportion of pork, with vegetables, bread, butter, ale or beer and cider, coffee and tea, all come in play and serve to restore the waste of tissue, and sustain the vigor of the body.

PROFESSIONAL MEN, THINKERS AND STUDENTS, whose expenditure is chiefly of the brain, and whose bodily activity is necessarily limited, require such a supply of nutriment as will measurably compensate for this waste. Hence, only a moderate supply of beef, mutton, lamb, ale or beer, but a larger proportion of fish, venison, wild or tame fowl, oysters, fruits, nuts, raisins or figs; and of the fish, trout, blue-fish, Spanish mackerel, or other game fish, are best; oat-meal in its various forms, wheaten grits, and coarse wheat bread, should form the staple of diet.

FOOD FOR FAT, CORPULENT PEOPLE.—In many families the tendency to corpulence and even obesity is constant. To many individuals it is the bane and dread of life. Yet such persons often use a diet directly tending to induce and aggravate the evil, while a proper diet always limits, and often removes the entire difficulty, for adipose tissue is only produced by certain fat-making articles of food. If these be avoided, the system may at the same time be nourished, and this accumulation of fat be prevented. The thanks of the world are due to MR. BANTING, an English gentleman, for having so clearly and forcibly elucidated this point in his pamphlet* on the subject, to which I refer those more particularly interested. I have had occasion to verify his observations in repeated instances. The fat-making articles are particularly butter, sugar, pork, milk, bread, potatoes, all sweet fruits, etc. Hence, the patient may eat all kinds of meat except pork—all kinds of fish except

*Banting, on corpulency.

salmon, all the fruits except those containing sugar in large proportion, and nearly all kinds of vegetables except potatoes. Now, by choosing a diet containing largely the articles allowed, and only a very little of well baked or toasted bread or potatoes, to which sour wine and tea and coffee may be added in moderation, and no butter, milk, or sugar, the most corpulent may reduce their weight several pounds per month, while improving their general health, strength and mental vigor. And this may be continued to any reasonable limit.

VERY LEAN, SPARE PEOPLE, by pursuing the opposite course, may increase their weight and embonpoint as well as their comfort. They should use sugar, milk, butter, bread, potatoes, pork, fat meat, oysters and fruits, figs, grapes and fish. These heat and fat-producing elements will, unless the assimilation be very faulty, soon produce a change for the better, which may be extended at the pleasure of the individual.

IN COLD WEATHER, when people are exposed to low temperatures, the more fat and heat-producing articles are required. Of these, pork, buckwheat, Indian corn, wheat bread, butter, milk, sugar, beer or ale, beans, peas, meat pies, poultry, etc., are among the more prominent.

IN WARM WEATHER the more cooling, less heat-producing articles are appropriate. The quantity of meat of any kind should be moderate, and that principally the lean of beef, lamb, veal or poultry, and well-ripened fruits of all kinds, and of vegetables in their seasons, with a due proportion of well-baked wheaten bread. Cooling drinks, acidulated with fruits, are in order and are very grateful and healthy.

A far more liberal and even generous use of fruits in their seasons, I am persuaded, would largely conduce to the health and welfare of our people.

THE DIET OF OLD PEOPLE should be regulated according to their individual condition. If they are fat, heavy and sleepy, inclined to sit and slumber, they should avoid fat meats, butter, sugar and fat-creating elements of food, and instead, eat of lean meat, brown bread, fish, nuts, fruits and vegetables, with the usual quantities of tea or coffee. On the contrary, if they are lean, irritable, querulous or sleepless, let them eat of fat meats, bread and butter, buckwheat cakes, rice, milk, potatoes, etc., and the better nourishment of the system will manifest itself in improved sleep, quiet and disposition.

## DIET OF THE SICK.

In general, sick people need but little food, but that which is given them should be nourishing and easily digested. During the progress of all acute diseases, fevers and inflammations especially, the process of digestion is mostly suspended, and nature indicates, by a want of appetite, bad taste, coated tongue, disgust or even loathing of food, the indisposition of the organism to receive or appropriate it. If food is forced upon the system at such times, it not only does no good, but injury, and no food can be of any value or afford nourishment to the system, unless it is digested. If the acute stage of disease is prolonged, the organism soon demands an amount of sustenance, equal to its daily waste, and then the discrimination of the nurse and attendants is required, so as to supply this waste without overtaxing the weak or exhausted digestive organs. Thus, during the acute or feverish stage of disease, water gruel, oat-meal gruel, toast water, barley water, pure water, weak black tea, and drinks made from any of the fresh or dried fruits, or orange water, or any ripe fruit, not too acid, are the usual and proper sustenance, and may be given in such quantities, and at such intervals, as the patient desires. After the more acute and feverish symptoms have passed over, the range may be enlarged, and milk toast, boiled rice, with a little sugar or butter, baked apples, fish and even ripe fruit are allowable.

In a condition of more advanced recovery or convalescence, beef tea, birds and small game, squirrels, rabbits, pigeons, and other game are in order, and tender steak, venison, lamb chops, fresh fish, oysters, clam soup, etc., may be proper. Where patients are exhausted or very low, beef tea, wine whey, wine and even brandy are proper and at times indispensable.

When patients are very feeble, and but little nourishment is given at a time, it may be given in comparative frequency, say once in two hours; usually, sick people may take a small meal as often as four or five times in the twenty-four hours. On the other hand, we should avoid feeding patients so frequently, as to keep the stomach in a state of constant repletion, and thus obliterate the faintly-returning desire for food.

During convalescence, the appetite revives and becomes sometimes ravenous, indicating a desire for abundant nourishing food, which may be gratified to any reasonable extent.

Weak black tea is allowable at all times, in a reasonable quantity, for the sick and convalescent. Tobacco should be used in moderation, if at all, while the patient is using Homeopathic medicine, and persons using it should always rinse the mouth thoroughly before taking the pills, and should refrain from smoking or chewing for an hour or more after having taken their medicine. Yet we find the moderate use of this narcotic far less prejudicial to the action of Homeopathic Medicine than has generally been supposed. Acids, spices, pepper, etc., in moderation, or used in the preparation of food, are not so objectionable as is usually held. Yet the system should not be deluged with the one or saturated with the other, if we expect a favorable action from Homeopathic treatment. The condiments used in preparing plain food, and the acids or mustard used in making a salad, need not be abandoned if used in moderation.

## EXERCISE.

Exercise is important to the invalid and those of sedentary habits; yet to be useful, it should be attended with pleasurable excitement and freedom from labor or anxious thought. In acute diseases, we are more inclined to exercise too much than too little, also in many chronic diseases. But in convalescence the patient should exercise either passively in a carriage, or by walking every day in the open air, limited only by the danger of exposure to cold, and his own strength and ability to sustain the effort. But if exercise exhausts one, excites vertigo, dizziness, or occasions pain, it will not prove beneficial. This is especially the case with sick or enfeebled persons, and may be considered a general rule.

## HOW TO SELECT, PREPARE AND TAKE THE MEDICINES.

In general, and for slight affections, after having first looked over or read the Manual, a glance at the indications on the inside cover of the case will be sufficient to show from what particular vial the medicine is to be taken for any particular disease or symptom. Yet if more than a single dose is required, it will be well to read over, in the Mentor, the description of the Disease or affection which is supposed to be present.

After having read the directions carefully, and selected the proper Specific, if the directions are to take the medicine dry, then take TWO of the pellets from the vial into the hand or a spoon, and thence into the mouth, and let them gradually dissolve without being chewed or swallowed whole like pills. It is a bad way to turn the vial against the tongue or into the mouth, as the breath contaminates and dissolves the pellets.

If it is designed to take several portions during the twenty-four hours, it is always best to take them in fluid form. For this purpose, count two pellets for every portion of medicine for an adult, or one pellet for young children, and putting these in a glass, add a tablespoonful of drinking water for each portion for an adult, or a teaspoonful for each portion for a child, and an extra spoonful for waste, and having crushed and dissolved them by stirring with the spoon, proceed to give according to the intervals mentioned.

Two Specifics may often be given in alternation, that is, first one, then after the proper interval, the other, and so on. Where specifics are to be thus given, let each be prepared according to the above directions, remembering that each glass has its separate spoon and label to prevent mixture or confusion.

This alternation of remedies is a favorite mode of treatment, and may be resorted to when all the symptoms do not seem to be met by one remedy, or when really two diseases may be present at the same time, as for instance: cough and fever, catarrh and dyspepsia, leucorrhœa and constipation, headache and dyspepsia. In such cases the two Specifics may be given alternately with advantage.

When we can do so, it is preferable to cure with a single Specific. In cases where some symptom does not seem to be within the range of the remedy, yet in using it a few days, this symptom or complaint often disappears with the main disease.

The best time for taking medicine is in the morning on rising and washing the mouth, and at night on retiring to rest.

## REPETITION OF DOSES.

The repetition of doses depends much upon circumstances. In acute diseases and in urgent cases, the Specific acts best when dissolved, and a spoonful given every fifteen minutes, half-hour, hour, two or four hours, according to the urgency of the case, always bearing in mind this rule, to *diminish the frequency of the doses in proportion as the patient improves,* and to discontinue the Specific altogether as soon as entire relief is afforded. In most cases of chronic disease, a dose morning and at night will be sufficient, or at most, three or four times a day. In very many cases a dose once per day is quite sufficient, and better than if more frequent. It is not the quantity or frequency of doses so much as the appropriateness of the remedy which cures the patient, and if a small quantity will not cure, there is but little hope of a large one.

# DISEASES AND TREATMENT.

## FEVERS.

Fevers have usually a precursory stage of some days, consisting of depression, pain in the limbs, headache, coated tongue, turns of vertigo, loss of appetite, or general lassitude. After this there is either a cold chill or chilliness for a day or two, which is followed by high fever, with headache, sleeplessness, often delirium, full, quick, hard pulse, quick respiration, vertigo on rising or sitting up, sometimes vomiting, costive bowels, etc.

This stage continues some days, depending upon the character of the fever and treatment, after which, in favorable terminations, the pulse by degrees abates, the skin gradually becomes moist, the tongue cleans off, appetite and strength improve, and the patient becomes convalescent.

### GENERAL RULES IN THE TREATMENT OF FEVERS.

Perfect rest of body and mind, freedom from care, annoyance and anxiety, as far as possible.

The room should be well ventilated, aired and lighted, and scrupulously clean.

The bed should be a hair mattress, or a quilt doubled on a straw or other bed, and the bed linen frequently aired and changed.

Pure cold water should be used as drink, and the face, hands and body should be frequently sponged off with tepid or cool water.

Toast water, gruel, barley or rice water may be used as drink after the fever has a little abated, or drink may be made of any mild, fresh or dried fruits, except when there is diarrhœa, when fruit drinks should be avoided.

Gradually a more substantial diet may be allowed, beginning with baked apples, boiled rice, toast bread, jellies, meat soups, clam soup, and yet more substantial articles of food during convalescence.

VARIETIES OF FEVER are not always sharply defined, and not unfrequently a fever assumes a particular character in its progress, or begins in one form and changes into another.

## ERETHIC OR SIMPLE FEVER.

It is usually transient, but may be the precursor of more serious disorders, and so demands attention.

It begins with a chill or shivering, which is succeeded by heat, thirst, general uneasiness, accelerated pulse and some prostration, and terminates in a profuse perspiration.

TREATMENT.—Give the Fever Specific, No. ONE, dissolved in water, as directed on page 52, a spoonful every half-hour during the violence of the chill and fever, and then as the heat and uneasiness abates and perspiration appears, give at intervals of an hour or more until entirely cooled off, and convalescence is established. This usually requires but a day or two, when the patient may be dismissed.

## INFLAMMATORY FEVER.

This form of fever commences with a chill of some duration, followed by high fever, strong, quick pulse, burning heat, red face, severe headache, hurried respiration, thirst, tossing and sleeplessness. The symptoms are worse in the evening and are better after midnight and towards morning. It may continue ten or fourteen days unless cut short by the Specific treatment, and if mismanaged by active cathartics, may readily run into typhus or typhoid, or other slow fevers.

It is caused by sudden check of perspiration, exposure to cold damp winds, intense mental emotions, high living, or mismanaged febrile attacks. It generally appears in persons of adult age, full habit and sanguine temperament.

TREATMENT.—In this form of fever only the FEVER SPECIFIC NO. ONE is required. Dissolve twenty pellets, in ten or twelve large spoonfuls of water in a glass; and of the fluid give a large spoonful every hour or even every half hour, at first, and so continue giving a spoonful at intervals of an hour or less during the height of the fever, and at longer intervals as the surface cools off and the surface grows moist, until the full crisis appears and the disease is subdued.

Sponge off the hands and face and even the surface of the body frequently during the dry, burning heat, and after sweating; and at first during the chill, or if the feet are inclined to be cold, or head very hot, a hot foot-bath will be of advantage. This treatment will generally promptly relieve and gradually arrest its progress. After the fever has subsided, the SPECIFIC NO. TEN, two pellets three times per day, should be given for some days, to complete the cure.

## BILIOUS OR GASTRIC FEVER, REMITTENT FEVER.

These fevers generally originate in some derangement of the stomach or digestive organs, or from malaria. In the origin and progress of the disease the derangement of the biliary or gastric system is prominent. It has less of the violent heat and inflammatory action than the fever so named, and yet not so much of nervous prostration and debility, as in typhoid fevers. The bilious form is more common in the Southern States, and in the hot season than in the more temperate regions, while the gastric fever is common in more Northerly regions.

It may be occasioned by great heat and excessive perspiration, which is suddenly checked, or by irritating substances taken into the stomach, or even by violent emotions such as anger, grief or care, or other excitement acting upon an irritable temperament, or in common with other causes.

SYMPTOMS.—It has a precursory stage, marked by decided gastric or biliary derangement, headache, coated tongue, bitter or foul taste, deficient appetite and general depression. After this there is a more or less prolonged chill, followed by sharp, pungent heat of the hands, face and surface, violent headache in the forehead, frequently delirium at night, sense of weight and fulness in the region of the stomach, nausea and inclination to vomit, belching up of wind, and vomiting of acid bile or of mucus mixed with bile, tongue thickly coated dirty yellow, bowels are frequently tender and at first constipated, afterwards tendency to diarrhœa. The face is pale and sickly, white of the eyes more or less yellow, pulse quick, tense, sometimes intermitting, and the urine is dark, cloudy, often thick and turbid. The more the liver is implicated, the more yellow the surface, the whites of the eyes, and the darker the urine and more yellow and thick coated the tongue.

The fever is subject to distinct remissions, coming on after a slight perspiration, and after some hours the fever recommences again and there may be a succession of these remissions, the more distinct they are, the more favorable for the patient. This fever is inclined to terminate in the intermittent form, or fever and ague.

TREATMENT.—The FEVER PILLS, NO. ONE and the BILIOUS PILLS, NO. TEN, are the proper remedies in this form of fever. Prepare according to directions on page 52, twelve or fourteen pellets of each number in separate glasses, and give for the first twelve hours, and until the force of the fever has somewhat abated, the FEVER PILLS, NO. ONE, a spoonful every hour. After that, give the two medicines, NO. ONE and NO. TEN, alternately, at intervals of one or two hours, according to the heat and intensity of the fever, and continue these until the violence of the disease is broken; then at longer intervals, until a cure is established.

Should a diarrhœa come on and threaten to become exhausting, suspend the use of the NO. TEN, and in place of it give the NO. FOUR, until the diarrhœa has abated, and then go on again as before.

Should the disease terminate in a regular INTERMITTENT FEVER, give the NO. SIXTEEN alternately with the NO. TEN every three hours, in solution, until the disease is cured.

In the invasive stage, before the fever has declared itself, two pellets of the NO. TEN, for indigestion, taken dry on the tongue two or three times a day, will correct the action of the stomach and liver, and arrest the entire disease.

## TYPHOID OR TYPHUS FEVERS

Are marked by great weakness and prostration of the system, fever usually not so high, but early delirium, dry or dark coated tongue, sleeplessness, or deep, profound sleep, pain in the head and back. This form of fever frequently commences with slight shiverings and dull heavy headache, oppression, anxious expression of the countenance, nausea, despondency and very drowsy or a quiet delirium, a slightly accelerated pulse, feeble and tremulous.

Sometimes the symptoms from the first assume a more pernicious form, beginning with alternations of chill and heat, with a tense hard pulse, sometimes quick, at others not increased in frequency; pain in the forehead and top of the head, and very generally in the back, sleeplessness and delirium at first, then low muttering delirium; putrid diarhœa, bleeding from the nose, and dark, putrid, or even bloody discharges from the bowels.

It is frequently caused, especially in its worst forms, by over-crowding, as upon shipboard or in work-houses or prisons, and hence deficient air and nutrition. Often overwork, exhaustion of body and mind, exposure and epidemic influences cause the milder forms of the disease. This form of fever generally attacks young or middle aged people, rarely children or the aged, and usually but once, the subject being thereafter exempt.

TREATMENT.—If a good Homeopathic Physician can be obtained, let him be called, if not proceed as follows: give the No. ONE and the No. SIXTEEN Specifics in alternation. Dissolve twelve or fourteen pellets in half as many large spoonfuls of water, each in separate glasses, and give alternately every two hours, first of No. ONE and then of No. SIXTEEN, as directed on page 52, and thus continue, being careful to have the room well ventilated, and have the hands, face and body frequently sponged off with tepid water during the heat.

When Typhus or Typhoid fever prevails in a family or vicinity, the use of the Specific, No. ONE, two pills morning and night, will protect the person from having the fever, a matter of much importance in some cases.

I do not advise the treatment of Typhoid, Typhus, or other severe forms of fevers, by non-professional persons. Circumstances may render it necessary, and hence the propriety of giving the treatment. But in general, such cases should be treated by a competent physician, as complications or changes may occur, for which no other person should assume the responsibility.

## FEVER AND AGUE.

This disease is so well known as scarcely to require remark. When fully developed, and of simple type, it consists of three stages—the cold stage or chill, the heat, and the sweating stage. During the chill there is usually pain in the head, back and limbs, nausea and even vomiting, thirst, blue nails, shivering, yawning, etc. During the heat, headache, sometimes delirium, hot skin, quick pulse, and other symptoms are usually present. This is usually followed by a profuse long-continued perspiration. The entire paroxysm, however, may be variously modified, as the hot and cold stage may be mixed, or the hot stage precede the cold, or the sweat be entirely wanting.

The paroxysm may return every day, every second day, or even at longer intervals, generally advancing an hour or two at each access, though sometimes postponing.

Directions.—As a Preventive: Persons residing where Fever and Ague is prevalent, or those traveling in such regions, along rivers, lowlands, plains, or marshes, may be protected from this disease by simply taking two of the Fever and Ague Pills, No. Sixteen every night on going to bed. If there are symptoms of its approach, such as depression, headache, bad taste in the mouth, chilliness and pain in the limbs: take two pills four times per day, and live for some days on very light, easily-digested diet, avoiding labor, over-work or fatigue.

To Cure the Disease: For chills which return *every day:* take two hours before each chill is to come on, four of the pills, permitting them to dissolve in the mouth; then take no medicine until the paroxysm is over and the sweat partially subsided, when four more pills are to be taken, and thus continue until the disease is broken. Then two pills every night and morning for four weeks, to prevent a relapse.

For chills which return *every other day:* take four pills one hour before each paroxysm comes on, and four more after it has passed off; then during the well day, take four pills morning, noon and night. In all other cases, take four pills, morning and night. In some cases, where the digestion seems much impaired and liver obstructed, the use of the No. Ten and the No. Sixteen, in alternation every three hours, has been promptly efficient in arresting the chills and curing the disease. After the chills have subsided, take four pills every night for four weeks, to prevent a return of the disease, and avoid exposure, heavy indigestible food, or severe labor. For children, give one-half as much medicine as for adults.

## DUMB AGUE, CHILL FEVER.

These are simply irregular forms of fever and ague, whose type has been broken by quinine, cholagogue or other drugs, or even by long continuance. The chill, heat and sweat are irregular or mixed; sometimes no chill, only long-continued heat, and at others only chill and long, lasting sweat.

Treatment.—Take the Fever and Ague Specific No. Sixteen, four pills three times per day, avoiding taking them during the paroxysm, but some little time before and afterwards.

## OLD SUPPRESSED AGUES.

The results of fever and ague, and the effects of quinine, arsenic, cholagogue, and other pernicious drugs so often used to suppress it, are often manifested by vertigo or turns of dizziness, ringing in the ears, deafness, enlarged spleen or ague-cake, swelling of the limbs or general dropsy, great feebleness and debility, coated tongue, weak digestion or liver complaint. In these bad complications the cure may require some time, but will be perfect and permanent.

Treatment.—This condition requires the use of the Fever and Ague Specific No. Sixteen, four pills morning and at night. Should the digestion be weak, two pills of No. Ten may also be taken each forenoon and afternoon. This course will prove promptly and permanently effectual.

## FEVERS OF CHILDREN.

Fevers among children of from one to ten years of age are quite common, and are often brought on by over fatigue, playing in the heat of the sun, exposure in light thin dress, or bare arms or legs to cold, chilly winds, improper food, sweetmeats, or the irritation of worms, provoked by such food, or the irritation of teething.

Such fevers are manifested by heat of the hands and surface, red face, or one cheek red and the other pale, swelling and throbbing of the veins of the neck, hot head, quick pulse, rapid breathing, fretfulness, and often inclination to sleep.

Treatment.—The Fever Specific, No. One is only required. Dissolve ten or twelve pellets in as many small spoonfuls of water, and of this give every half-hour at first, and then every hour, a spoonful, until the disease is subdued. Should the fever have been occasioned by indigestible substances—raisins, oranges or sweetmeats—and the bowels be constipated, give an injection of tepid salt and water, and repeat it if necessary. And should there be twitchings and startings on going to sleep, thus indicating convulsions, give two pills of the Specifie for convulsions, No. THIRTY-THREE, and repeat it again after two or three hours if necessary. Drink moderately of water, and often sponge off the body with tepid water. Keep them on very low diet and quiet until relieved. This is the proper treatment for all forms of fevers and even inflammation in children.

## SCARLET FEVER; SCARLATINA.

This is usually considered a very formidable disease, but under the mild and efficient system of Homeopathic treatment, it has lost most of its terrors. True, sometimes an epidemic may pass over the country, of unusual violence which carries off quite a proportion of its little sufferers, but in general, it passes as a comparatively mild and harmless disease.

There are some three varieties, marking, in fact, degrees in the severity of the disease, and the degree of danger likely to attend it.

In the SIMPLE FORM, it commences with peevishness, chilliness, headache, nausea and vomiting, after which the eruption appears, first at the face and upper extremities and subsequently over the body, either diffused or in patches, assuming a bright scarlet color, breath offensive, tongue coated, high fever and soreness of the throat.

The ANGINOSE variety has more violent symptoms, commences with vomiting, which may continue for hours, high fever, quick pulse, eruption somewhat paler and in patches or diffused; the tonsils become inflamed and swelled, and ulcerate; tongue dirty-white or red, great prostration; after some days swelling of the glands of the cheek and beneath the ear; the fever is very high, and surface hot and dry, and often discharge of hot excoriating mucus from the nose.

In the MALIGNANT form, the most violent symptoms are manifested about the head, and it sometimes terminates in fatal congestion before the eruption has fully made its appearance; in milder cases there is constant vomiting, violent pain in the head, stupor with half-closed eyes, pale imperfect eruption in spots or of brick-dust color, and after these excoriating discharge from the nose.

In the milder forms the eruption should begin to grow pale and disappear in three or four days, and the fever and sore throat abate, and the child be well in a week. But the other varieties are uncertain, and may require ten or fourteen days, or even longer for a cure.

You may recognize the scarlet fever from other diseases by the vomiting, the sore throat, the high fever, and the subsequent eruption.

TREATMENT.—As a preventive, when scarlet fever prevails in the neighborhood, give the children each morning and night one of the FEVER PILLS NO. ONE.

So soon as the vomiting or fever has declared itself, commence with the FEVER SPECIFIC NO. ONE, dissolved in water, twelve pellets in as many teaspoonsful of water, of which give a spoonful every hour. Continue this from day to day, preparing new medicine daily, except when the patient is quietly sleeping at the time for giving the medicine, then give it after the patient awakes.

For the vomiting, if severe or frequent, interpose two pellets of Specific NO. SIX, and repeat it two or three times in alternation with the NO. ONE, until the vomiting is relieved.

After two or three days it will be best to alternate Specific NO. FOURTEEN with NO. ONE, prepared in like man-

5

ner, and give the two medicines at intervals of two hours, and so continue until the disease is cured.

Should there occur swellings under the ear or jaw, if the fever has gone, give the Specific No. TWENTY-THREE in alternation with No. FOURTEEN. If discharges from the ear or earache, give the No. TWENTY-TWO instead. If dropsical swellings, which sometimes occur in consequence of taking cold, the No. TWENTY-FIVE, two pills three times per day, will soon relieve.

## MEASLES.

Measles prevail usually towards spring, and is generally a mild, easily-managed disease. It commences with symptoms of bad cold, sneezing, lachrymation, and slight redness of the eyes, and soon a hoarse, *loose* cough, which is characteristic of the disease. The rash appears first on the face in minute pimples in clusters, with a reddish blush, deepening and increasing as it comes out—the first day upon the face and neck, next upon the body, and the third day extending to the lower extremities, by which time it grows fainter upon the face, and disappears in the same manner. There is fever, loose cough, hoarseness, etc.

TREATMENT.—Give the Fever Specific No. ONE, prepared as directed on page 52, every two hours, and continue this treatment through the entire course of the disease. If the measles do not *come out well*, do not be alarmed about that; keep the patient warm, give some warm tea or nourishing soup, a hot foot-bath, but nothing else; the measles will come out sufficiently. If the cough is troublesome, alternate the Cough Pills No. SEVEN with the No. ONE. If very hoarse, give a few doses of the Croup Pills. If the eyes are at all red, inflamed, intolerant of light, the No. EIGHTEEN will be found to act like a charm, given in alternation with No. ONE, and for any weakness of sight remaining or in consequence of measles, they may be relied upon, giving two pills morning and night. Care should be taken during the measles, to prevent taking cold, as serious diseases of the lungs may arise as a consequence.

## SMALL-POX; VARIOLOID.

Small-pox and its modified form, termed varioloid, is a strictly infectious disease, being always communicated by contagious matter or effluvia from those who have it. It is important to recognize it at the earliest hour possible, in order to adopt a proper treatment as well as to prevent others from exposure. These circumstances will aid us in establishing the diagnosis. The disease comes on in from nine to fourteen days after exposure. It begins with chilliness, some fever, a peculiar swimming or dizziness of the head and headache, pain in the back, often quite severe and constant, derangement of the stomach, often nausea and vomiting, aching in the bones and soreness of the flesh, and among children and in violent cases, it is ushered in by violent convulsions.

After the symptoms above have continued three days, the ERUPTION begins to come out, showing itself first on the forehead and face in the form of minute red points, which increase in size from day to day, while others make their appearance on the face and by degrees over the hands, arms and other portions of the body, but always more numerous on the forehead and face. If the face is red and swelled, it will be likely to assume the *confluent* form, the pustules all running together and forming a complete crust. But if the face is but little swelled or pale, the pock coming out scattered only here and there, the disease will assume the *discreet* form, with only a few pustules that fill; the fever, vertigo, headache and pains pretty much disappearing as the pock comes out and the disease running a mild course. After four days of development, during which the pustules attain their growth, the *suppurative stage* commences, during which the pock become filled with a yellowish fluid, which gradually changes to a turbid appearance, each pock surrounded by a red circle with a dark indentation at the top. About the tenth or eleventh day from the commencement and towards the close of this stage, there is for two or three days considerable fever and flow of saliva; after this has passed the pustules gradually grow brownish, dry up and fall off, leaving cicatrixes or marks of a deep red color, which are quite a period in assuming the natural color of the skin.

TREATMENT.—This disease under Homeopathic treatment, is more loathsome than dangerous, and properly treated and understood, generally passes off as a mild, though unpleasant visitation. Two points are of especial consideration, especially during the earlier stages of the disease, namely: To KEEP THE PATIENT COOL, with at all times plenty of fresh air. As soon as the nature of the disease is understood, *keep the room entirely cool, give no warm teas or heating drinks,* and thus prevent the formation of numerous pock, the less of which the better. Children attacked with convulsions should be taken at once into the open air or a room without fire for relief.

All through the disease the greatest possible cleanliness should be observed, with frequent change of linen. When the pustules begin to form, the room should be darkened, which is a partial security against the pitting from the disease. Give only cold water, cold toast-water or black tea cold for drink. Gruel of meal, oat-meal, barley, rice or farina, all taken cold, is the best nourishment. After the disease has spent its force, baked apples, boiled rice, custard, toast, etc., may be allowed.

As medicines, from the first symptoms, give the Specific

No. ONE, twelve pellets in water as directed on page 52, of which give a spoonful every hour during the entire presence of fever. After the fever has measurably abated, prepare the Specific No. FOURTEEN in like manner with No. ONE, and give the two alternately at two hours intervals, until the drying off of the crusts.

P. S.—If the SARRACENIA PURPUREA can be procured, give it from the first and all through the disease: ten drops of the tincture in a glass half-full of water, which give in spoonful doses alternately with the No. ONE. I have known it to arrest the disease when given early, and to materially shorten its course and prevent the pitting.

## PREVENTION OF SMALL-POX.

There is unquestionably some risk in vaccination. Matter from an unhealthy subject may be introduced, carrying disease with it, and thus life-long evils be inflicted. But these results are not common, and the careless abuse of a system, rather than its legitimate use. Matter should be selected with care, from a healthy child, one who has no scrofulous or syphilitic taint in its system, and has no eruption of any kind upon the skin or scalp. Matter taken from such a subject, introduced just beneath the skin of the outside of the upper third of the left arm, inserted not so deep as to make it bleed, and yet deep enough to show a slight discoloration, will run a mild course, produce a pustule in ten or fourteen days, that in drying, will give a tamarind-stone like crust, and leave a deep and peculiar cicatrix which will show during a life time. If during the course of the vaccination any fever should manifest itself, give the Specific No. ONE, and if any eruption of the surface, give Specific No. FOURTEEN, night and morning, until it disappears.

After many years of observation, and balancing all the

dangers and inconvenience of vaccination and non-vaccination, my conclusion is, that every child should be vaccinated, and adults may be properly re-vaccinated when in danger of exposure to immediate contagion. This is the shortest, safest and best method.

## CHICKEN POX.

This disease has sometimes been confounded with small-pox or varioloid. But it may be known by the vesicles appearing mostly on the covered parts of the body or scalp, while in small-pox, they are mostly in the face, by the vesicles being smooth and transparent, filled with water and growing rapidly, attaining the size of a pea in a day; while in small-pox they are pustules firm and hard, begin to fill only after three or four days of growth. With chicken pox there is some fever, the thin watery vesicles come out often in clusters, commence with a thin pellicle which burst or dry up, forming a small puckered scab and rarely leaves a pit or depression.

The whole disease is mild, and usually runs its course in four or five days, unattended with danger.

TREATMENT.—Give the Specific No. ONE, ten pellets dissolved in as many spoonfuls of water, of which give a spoonful every one or two hours during the course of the disease. If a new crop of vesicles comes out afterwards, give two pellets of the Specific No. FOURTEEN, morning and night, until the case is cured.

## MUMPS.

This disease consists of a swelling of the salivary glands, and is usually not dangerous unless the patient is exposed to cold during the progress of the disease, and it makes a transition (metastasis) to some other organ. It is usually known as a swelling of the parotid gland in front of, and beneath the ear, first commencing on one side and then extending to the other, rarely both at once; sometimes the whole neck is involved and the swelling extends beneath the jaw. It is attended with fever, *and pain when chewing*, especially firm or hard food, and sometimes pain in swallowing. Sometimes the fifth or seventh day, the swelling leaves the neck and attacks the breasts or testicles, which become red, swelled and painful. At times, in sensitive children with prominent heads, it has been known to fall upon the brain, producing delirium or other dangerous symptoms.

TREATMENT.—Keep the child in a comfortable warm room, prevent exposure, make no applications except a light cloth around the neck and give no stimulants. Give the Specific No. ONE, ten pellets dissolved in as many spoonfuls of water, of which give one every hour. After the fever has abated, prepare the Specific No. TWENTY-THREE in like manner, and give alternately with No. ONE, at intervals of two hours, until the disease has disappeared. Should the disease fall upon the testicle, the Specific No. THIRTY will soon relieve, given every two or three hours. For fever, delirium or congestion to the head, the No. ONE is perfectly appropriate and will soon relieve.

## WHOOPING-COUGH.

This disease usually prevails as an epidemic and is supposed to be contagious. Persons are rarely attacked but once, and generally in childhood. Under our mild system of treatment it generally runs a mild course in from two to six weeks, while left to itself or under old school treatment, it may continue from ten to twelve weeks, and is often a most serious and not unfrequently fatal disease.

It usually commences as a common cold, though from the first the cough is more spasmodic and convulsive than from a catarrh. After a week or two the cough assumes its true distinctive character, which consists *in a rapid succession of shocks or coughs, succeeded by a long drawn, deep inhalation or whoop.* It is generally attended with some degree of fever, and, after it has reached its acme and began to decline, there is at the conclusion of each cough, expectoration of a quantity of thick gluey mucus. In some instances, vomiting occurs with almost every violent cough, and the little sufferer seems to be able to retain but little food, and with nervous children, convulsion or stiffening of the body and limbs, and loss of breath are not uncommon. At times the cough is so violent that blood is forcibly thrown from the nose and mouth, and the whites of the eyes become injected or suffused with blood. The disease becomes dangerous when the inflammation attacks the mucus membrane or substance of the lungs, thus producing a complicated pneumonia or bronchitis. When this occurs, the cough loses its convulsive character, becomes short and dry, with high fever and short labored respiration. These complications or severe symptoms are rare under our system of treatment.

TREATMENT.—TO PREVENT THE WHOOPING COUGH, when children have been exposed to it or begin to cough, simply give of the Specific NO. TWENTY, one pill three times per day, and the result will be that the cough will disappear or pass off as a mild non-convulsive catarrhal cough.

TREATMENT.—TO CURE THE DISEASE: Give of the Specific NO. TWENTY, one pill four times per day, for children under two years of age, and two pills at a time for those older, either dry, or in water, as may be most convenient, and continue this through the entire course of the disease.

If at any time *fever* should manifest itself, or the cough become dry and harsh, dissolve eight pellets of Specific No.

ONE, in eight teaspoonfuls of water, of which give a spoonful every one or two hours, intermediate with Specific No. TWENTY, and continue this until the fever abates, and the cough becomes soft and moist.

Let the child live on light diet, little or no meat, cake, pastry, or rich, or heavy food, but an abundance of *mucilaginous drinks,* rice water, barley water, gum water, or even weak black tea, or chocolate.

# DISEASES OF THE SKIN.

It has been common to treat all kinds of eruptions by means of applications directly to the surface, which is the particular seat of the disease. But the human system being a unit, it follows, of necessity, that no eruption can form upon the surface without the co-existence of a certain morbid condition of the system. Hence the propriety of treating all such eruptions with internal remedies alone, and hence the brilliant results which have attended such a method of treatment. It is often not difficult to repel an eruption from the surface by medicinal applications. But the disease is usually not only not cured, but merely repelled, to fall upon some other organ or surface, and is generally as much worse than the former condition, as its new location is more unnatural and more difficult to heal. Hence, for all such forms of disease, we prescribe nothing for the surface involved beyond the proper purity and cleanliness, and merely advise the internal use of our remedy for such forms of disease. A cure will then result naturally, permanently, and without injury to the system.

## ERYSIPELAS, ROSE.

This disease assumes two or three distinct forms, and though sometimes trivial, is oftentimes a very serious disease. The acute form commonly appears on the face, commencing on one cheek, or ear, or under the eye, as a deep reddish blush, with swelling of the part, and from thence extending over the face, and often the scalp, like a fire, attended with redness, swelling, itching, heat and burning of the part, and followed by desquamation or scaling off of the surface, over which the erysipelas has passed. Often blisters or vesicles arise, filled with yellow serum, which burst, covering the surface with a thickish crust. There is considerable fever, and when the erysipelas assumes the phlegmonous form, the inflammation not only involves the skin, but the tissue beneath it, and deep ulcerations and formation of matter are very liable to occur. This is more particularly the result, when the erysipelas attacks a limb, arm, leg, foot or hand. When erysipelas of the face occurs, and the affection is attended with high fever, and extends and spreads over the scalp, the brain is apt to become affected, attended with delirium, dread of light, and other very grave symptoms. Happily, under our mild system of treatment, such terminations are unusual, and the disease generally passes off as a very mild affair.

Sometimes a part is injured even very slightly, and owing to mismanagement or a peculiar condition of the system, an erysipelatious inflammation sets in, which assumes a very grave and dangerous character, and requires careful management.

Treatment.—From the first, the Specific No. Fourteen is the proper remedy, not only for light and trivial cases, but for those of the gravest character. Dissolve twelve pellets in six large spoonfuls of water, of which give to children a small, and to adults a large spoonful, every two hours, and continue this treatment without interruption during the waking hours. In acute erysipelas, or when there is fever, or in erysipelas of the face, or when there is tendency to assume a severe or malignant form, prepare also the Specific No. One, in the same manner as No. Fourteen, and give the two in alternation, at intervals of one hour, and to continue the use of No. One until the fever, heat, and swelling is allayed, when the cure may be finished with No. Fourteen. No application should be made to the surface; grease or oily substances and water are pernicious; scorched flour sometimes allays the itching; and the patient should live on very light diet, no meat or meat soups until full convalescence.

Erysipelas of the legs often appears in a very torpid form, as a *darkish red or mottled patch* on the leg, without fever or much heat or irritation of the part, and aside from the discoloration, the patient would scarcely know of its existence. In these cases, give the Specific No. Fourteen, two pills four times per day, dry or dissolved, live on light diet and rest the limbs as much as possible, and the disease will disappear.

## ZONA OR SHINGLES.

This is a form intermediate between herpes and erysipelas, and quite common. It comes out on some portion of the body, generally between the shoulders and hips, in the form of a belt, usually about a hand's breadth, and extending around a portion of the body. The eruption consists of small vesicles or blisters upon this reddish inflamed basis, and attended with burning, stinging and itching. It is frequently attended with fever. It arises from the same causes as erysipelas and requires the same treatment, and is rarely dangerous.

Treatment.—Give the Specific No. Fourteen, two pills every two or three hours, and if there is fever, alternate the Specific No. One with it, as an intermediate remedy. It will disappear in two or three days.

## NETTLE RASH, URTICARIA, HIVES.

This affection mostly attacks children, though some adults have it in a diffused form with much severity.

It generally appears as a feverless eruption, coming out in spots much like the sting of a bee or mosquito, or the sting of nettles, a pale, or red, or whitish eminence, somewhat hard, from half an inch to an inch in diameter, often clustered together; these spots are attended with heat, itching and burning, causing great annoyance. They disappear after some hours, and reappear again in other locations, being more likely to appear in cool, than in warm temperature. In adults, it sometimes appears as a deep scarlet rash, attended with heat, itching and swelling, and covering the entire person. It is usually developed by changes of temperature, over-eating, or eating certain kinds of fish or shell fish, and in children is almost always connected with some derangement of the digestion. It is apt to reappear from time to time.

TREATMENT.—Give the Specific No. FOURTEEN, two pellets morning, noon and night. This will be sufficient in ordinary cases. But if there is considerable of it on the person, arms or limbs, or fever, and the itching is annoying, dissolve eight or ten pellets of Specific No. ONE, in as many spoonfuls of water, of which give one every hour until relieved, then trust for the cure to No. FOURTEEN, given three times per day.

In chronic cases and to eradicate it from the system, and when the digestion is at fault, give two pellets of No. FOURTEEN, morning and noon, and two pellets of Specific No. TEN, at night.

## CHILBLAINS.

This affection is often troublesome in the winter, or in cold frosty weather. It is a sort of chronic erysipelas, being roused into activity from the effects of cold and change of temperature. It mostly makes its appearance along the sides of the feet, the soles and heels, in the form of small pea-size lumps, often reddish, attended with violent itching and burning, when in the warmth of the room. Sometimes the affection extends to the fingers, hands, ears and nose, and in very bad cases the chilblains have been known to burst, leaving very deep and ugly sores. Chilblains are often the result of having frost bitten the part, though they are always connected with some dyscrasia of the system. They disappear in summer but are apt to return very regularly in cold weather.

TREATMENT.—Dissolve ten or twelve pellets of Specific No. ONE, in as many spoonfuls of water, of which give every hour to children a tea, and to adults a large spoonful until the itching and irritation are relieved. Then give of Specific No. FOURTEEN, two pellets three times per day, to complete the cure.

Bathe the parts with WITCH HAZEL, to be obtained at the shops. It will promptly relieve the burning and irritation, and may be used in conjunction with the other Specifics named.

## FROST BITES AND FROZEN LIMBS.

When any portion of the person has been frost bitten or frozen, the part, ear, nose, cheek, fingers or toes, should immediately be rubbed in snow or ice cold water, and this should be carefully continued until the part becomes red and the sensation and circulation are restored. Then the best application is WITCH HAZEL. Moisten a fine rag or some cotton batting with the same, and envelop the frost bitten part with it, and then from time to time remoisten and apply it, as it gets dry, until the part is restored. Specific No. FOURTEEN, two pills four times per day, will aid in restoring the part.

## RING-WORM; HERPES CIRCINNATUS.

This is a form of herpes that is quite common, usually commencing in a spot and thence spreading out in a circular form, and as the centre regains its natural appearance, and the borders extend, it forms a ring—hence the name. At times rings form within each other, and extend in broken or imperfect forms, in various directions. The ring is occupied by small vesicles, which after some days break and leave a rough, reddish surface, with a rose-colored base. The rings appear upon the face, shoulder, arms, hands, in fact upon any part of the body. The duration of the disease is uncertain. It may continue a long time as successive crops of rings are produced, and it has been supposed to be contagious, from the fact, that several children, in the same school, or persons in the same family, are found to have it at the same time.

TREATMENT.—The Specific No. FOURTEEN is the appropriate remedy. Give two pellets three or four times per day, either dry or in water, and the affection will soon disappear.

## SCALD HEAD; TENIA CAPITIS; PORRIGO.

This disease may appear in different forms, and is always contagious, being readily communicated from one child to another, by means of the comb, brush, towel or even by contact of the diseased part. It is one of the most obstinate of eruptions, and very serious consequences inevitably result from repelling it from the surface, by means of ointments, or other external applications. It usually commences as a cluster of minute vesicles or pimples, in colored, irregular, circular patches, on which appear yellow points or patches, which contain a yellowish-white, thick, viscid fluid, of an offensive odor. This discharge is corrosive and irritates the surface, causing the eruption to extend. The hair becomes glued up and matted, and thick hard elevated crusts are formed of varied shape and appearance. This form of tenia is most liable to commence at the back of the head, towards the nape of the neck, and swelling and enlargement of the glands of the neck are not unusual.

Sometimes this disease appears as a dry scurfy eruption, cutting off the hairs of the head like a knife, and leaving bald, rough, scurfy spots, or patches. The first form at times in impoverished, neglected subjects, becomes complicated with some dyscrasia of the system, and the entire scalp becomes covered with large pustules, discharging a yellow or greenish fetid ichorous fluid, which gums up the entire hair of the scalp like a cap of pitch, the humor drying and forming thick, hard, coherent greyish-green crusts, and covering ulcers of considerable dimensions.

TREATMENT.—The less moisture, water, soap-suds, etc. is applied to the scalp the better. Water and soap, while they soften and cleanse the part, seem to convey the infection to the healthy portion of the scalp, while the effect upon the diseased point is not very beneficial. Hence, keep the head as clean as possible, and use as little water or soap as possible, shingle off the hair over the diseased parts, or the entire head at once, the sooner the better.

Give the Specific No. FOURTEEN, two pills dissolved in a spoonful of water, three or four times per day. The diet should be mild and not exciting. Should there be heat and irritation of the scalp, an occasional portion of two pellets of Specific No. ONE may be given with advantage.

## CRUSTA SERPEGINOSA.

This is a severe and inveterate affection of the skin, very liable to become chronic, and to be attended with swellings of the glands, of the groin, and axilla.

It commences with a red itching spot on the cheek, in

front of the ear, upon which small dark pimples arise, which itch violently, and the spot becomes surrounded with a bright red halo. These vesicles break and exude a quantity of serous, corroding fluid, which causes the infant to scratch continually, and excites new eruption wherever it extends. In this manner the affection extends over the face, eyelids, and sometimes the hairy scalp. As the disease progresses the eruption sometimes makes its appearance on the neck, back, loins, and extremities, even after the disease has left the face. The fluid exuded from the eruption, later becomes hardened, assuming the form of small, flat, dark crusts, which become detached by the newly formed matter, and leave a sore, ichorous place in the skin. The itching causes constant restlessness, sleeplessness, general debility, and loss of flesh; the infant becoming visibly emaciated. The glands of the axilla and groin frequently become affected, swell and sometimes even suppurate, leaving unpleasant abscesses, and in grown persons, abscesses form on different parts of the trunk or extremities, which attain the size of a walnut, break and leave bluish spots on the skin.

TREATMENT.—The Specific No. FOURTEEN is the proper remedy and should be given, two pills four times per day, for one week, dissolving each portion in a teaspoonful of water, or give them dry if the disease is only slight. After the No. FOURTEEN has thus been given one week, the doses may be reduced to one at noon, and one at night, and two pellets of Specific No. TWENTY-TWO should be given each morning. If there is violent itching, redness, and burning, and intolerable restlessness of the child, dissolve six pellets of Specific No. ONE in six spoonfuls of water, and give a spoonful every hour, until the itching abates, and rest is procured. This is the proper treatment, and should be persevered in until the disease is cured.

## ITCH-SCABIES.

This well known disease consists of a peculiar eruption of the skin, characterized by pointed vesicles, usually small, transparent at the top, and filled with thin matter, and sometimes these pimples become enlarged to pea size, like pustules or blisters. The pimples on being scratched, often bleed freely, or the tops become filled with dark blood. The eruptions appear on every part of the body, except the face, generally most abundant on the wrists, and between the fingers, less so on the arms, and legs, and body. It is attended with violent itching, worse at night and when undressing, and is more common and more likely to appear on children then adults. It is strictly infectious and readily communicated by contact, clothing, or sleeping in the same bed.

Treatment.—This is not a disease to be cured in a day. It will at best require some weeks, if fully developed, ofttimes longer. The patient should have plain, but good wholesome food, free from condiments or stimulants as possible, and the greatest care should be observed by frequent bathing, and change of linen, to keep the skin as pure and free from infectious matter as possible. Prepare likewise a lotion, by putting one ounce flour of sulphur to eight ounces of alcohol, and after shaking well, put a tablespoonful of this tincture to a coffee cup of water, and after bathing every night, apply this to the surface.

Dissolve daily eight pellets of Specific No. Fourteen in four spoonfuls of water, of which give a spoonful four times per day until cured. Better than even this is the *Sulphur Soap*, which may be procured at the Druggists. This may be applied at night after bathing, forming a lather upon the surface which may be sponged off the next morning.

## BOILS, FERUNCLES.

Boils are well known as tumors, somewhat conical in shape, which are hard, inflame slowly, suppurate and discharge. The matter first discharged is bloody or mixed with blood, but afterwards is pus or altered tissue, and at last in a hard mass termed a *core*. Not unfrequently boils appear successively or in crops upon the same individual, continuing for months, and causing great annoyance and suffering.

TREATMENT.—The Specifics No. ONE and No. THIRTY-FIVE should be given in alternation, four or six pellets of each dissolved in as many spoonfuls of water, and taken in alternation two or four times a day, according to the urgency of the case. A cloth wet in diluted WITCH HAZEL and laid on the boil will soon allay the pain and inflammation, or diluted arnica may answer the same purpose.

To prevent a recurrence of the boil, or a new crop, take for two or three weeks, two pellets of No. FOURTEEN at night, and of No. THIRTY-FIVE each morning.

## CARBUNCLE; ANTHRAX.

The carbuncle differs from the boil, though somewhat similar. It is a deep seated, hard circumscribed swelling, of livid hue, attended with great pain, itching, and burning heat. It does not suppurate and discharge like the boil, but a thin acrid offensive fluid runs from several openings which communicate with each other, leaving for a time a whitish mass within, which, in being discharged, leaves a deep, ugly cavity.

The disease runs its course slowly, is attended with fever and prostration, and when the tumor is large, and seated on the head, spine or nape, is not free from danger.

TREATMENT.—At first, while there is considerable fever, the Specific No. ONE should be given hourly in fluid, and after the fever has abated, and the tumor more advanced, the Specifics No. TWENTY-TWO and No. TWENTY-THREE should be given in alternation every two hours. Dissolve eight pellets of each, in four spoonfuls of water, in separate glasses, and give every three hours a spoonful alternately. An application of diluted WITCH HAZEL, or arnica diluted, will be of some relief, or a poultice of flax seed, where the tumor is very hard, hot and unyielding. The medicinal influence is the main relief. and the disease at best yields slowly.

## WHITLOW, OR FELON.

This is an affection which usually appears at the end of the finger, sometimes around the roots of the nail, and at others, down deep beneath the fascia, or in the ball of the finger or thumb. It is usually attended with heat, swelling, and great pain, and is liable to reappear in the same person, unless the proper constitutional Homeopathic remedies are used to eradicate the predisposition from the system.

TREATMENT.—The Specific No. TWENTY-TWO is the proper remedy, of which dissolve twelve pellets in six spoonfuls of water, and give a spoonful every two or three hours, continuing the same from day to day. Poultices of flax seed, slippery elm, or bread and milk, may be applied with advantage, to soften the swelling and hasten suppuration, and the matter had best be discharged as soon as fluctuation is clearly perceived.

## ABSCESSES.

The term abscess is usually employed to indicate any morbid collection of matter.

There are in general two kinds of abscesses, the ACUTE and the CHRONIC. THE ACUTE is always preceded by soreness or sensibility of the part, followed by suppuration. The appearance of the skin changes with the commencement of suppuration. The surface, usually red, becomes livid, the pain becomes more dull and throbbing, the swelling increases in bulk, and if not too deeply seated, fluctuation may be discovered, and at this time there are almost always more or less of chills or slight rigors, succeeded by heat. After the abscess is fully ripe it assumes a more conical form or is said to point, and over this space the skin becomes livid, yellowish, and ere long bursts and the contents are discharged.

CHRONIC abscesses often begin and approach the surface, without any considerable constitutional disturbance, and the discharge is unhealthy, thin, serous, and containing flaky or cheesy substances. If the abscess is large, after the pus is evacuated and air admitted, the surrounding cyst becomes inflamed, and severe constitutional disturbance, hectic fever, etc., may arise.

TREATMENT.—We may hasten the suppurative process of acute abscesses, by applying warm poultices or fomentations, and they likewise afford some relief.

After the formation of matter is clearly announced by fluctuation, and the pointing or protrusion of some portion of the abscess, the matter should be discharged by a lancet inserted at the most depending portion of the abscess, and if the collection of matter is large, it may be necessary to repeat the process.

The Specifics No. ONE and No. TWENTY-TWO should be given alternately, every two or three hours, during the inflammatory stage, and until suppuration occurs. Then omit the No. ONE, and in place give the No. TWENTY-THREE, and so continue the Nos. TWENTY-TWO and TWENTY-THREE, at intervals of three or four hours, until the abscess is healed.

For CHRONIC abscesses, the Nos. TWENTY-TWO and

TWENTY-THREE should be given, two pellets in water, and four times per day in alternation.

## CORNS.

These troublesome excrescences are far more liable to form on the feet of some persons than others, thereby showing a constitutional predisposition, which is a proper subject of medical treatment. Tight shoes, the constant pressure upon some part of the foot, commonly give occasion to their formation, and hence frequent change of boots or shoes are of advantage. It is far from wise to constantly wear the same covering for the feet. Heavy thick boots or shoes for winter and wet weather, Arctic rubbers for snow and severe cold, light shoes for summer, and slippers for evening and house wear. This variety of covering is not only suitable and comfortable, but relieve the feet from constant pressure on the same or suffering parts, and withal are economical.

TREATMENT.—When corns or bunions are inflamed and troublesome, soak the feet well in warm water at night, and pare down the corn and take out the chit or hard core in the centre, and, after wiping the feet, apply WITCH HAZEL freely, following the bathing up for several nights. The relief will be prompt.

Besides, take of the Specific No. TWENTY-TWO, two pellets each night, and of No. THIRTY-FIVE, two pellets each morning for a week or more, to break up the predisposition to their formation.

# DISEASES OF THE HEAD AND NERVOUS SYSTEM.

---

## HEADACHES.

*Headaches* are various in their character and are produced by a variety of causes. It is less frequently a disease itself, than a symptom of some more general affection. Sometimes it is comparatively trivial, at other times of very grave importance, often interrupting any constant avocation of the patient, causing great suffering, and prostrating the system so frequently as to rapidly undermine the general health. With some persons, the slightest indiscretion in diet, or deviation from ordinary quiet habits, is followed by an attack of headache. The pain may be located in a single part, or involve the entire head; and is often accompanied with extreme nausea and painful retching and vomiting. The attacks are often provoked by some exposure, excitement, or error in diet, and sometimes they return at pretty regular intervals of seven or fourteen days. They may likewise be of congestive, rheumatic, bilious, catarrhal, or nervous origin.

Congestive headaches occur in plethoric persons of full habit, and are accompanied by a sense of fulness and throbbing in the head, red or very pale face, redness of the eyes, with sense of soreness on turning them, and often intolerance of light.

In bilious headache there is often coated tongue, bad taste in the mouth, and the pain is dull, aching or racking, sometimes moving from one part to the other, while the scalp may be sore and bowels constipated. Catarrhal headaches are indicated by dull, heavy pains across the forehead and upper part of the nose, attended with obstruction of the nose or fluent discharges.

TREATMENT.—Persons who are subject to headaches, should abandon the use of coffee, and also of strong tea, as the use of these beverages often contribute to keep up the disease, and in some cases alone cause it. They should live regularly and temperately, and avoid as far as possible, the known or exciting causes of the disease. Beside this regimen, they should take each morning two pellets of Specific No. THIRTY-FIVE, and at night two more of Specific No. TEN, as a preventive, and to eradicate the predisposition to these attacks.

When a paroxysm of headache comes on, if it has the symptoms of congestion mentioned above, the Specifics No. ONE and No. THIRTY-FIVE should be given every hour, alternately.

If the attack indicates a bilious condition, the Specifics No. NINE and No. TEN should be given every hour in alternation, two pellets at a dose. Should the attack commence with blindness, soon followed by nausea and vomiting, or other severe symptoms, the medicines are best when dissolved in water, and given every half hour, or even more frequently. Should there be heat, fever or throbbing of the vessels of the head or temples, substitute the Specific No. ONE for the No. TEN, and continue in the same manner.

For the usual form of SICK-HEADACHE, as it is generally termed, with nausea, vomiting, prostration, often intolerance of light or noise, the Specifics Nos. NINE and TEN should be given every hour or half hour, in alternation, until relieved.

*Headaches in Females,* occuring just before or during the monthly period, will be relieved by taking the Specific No. ELEVEN, either alone or in alternation with No. THIRTY-

FIVE, especially if the periods are painful or too profuse. Headaches from constipation will be cured by using the Specific No. TEN, two pellets night and morning.

The cure of old, long-standing headaches requires time and perseverance, but can always be accomplished by the persevering use of the Specifics before mentioned.

Persons subject to headaches, find, on arising with the symptoms of a headache in the morning, or at other times, that by taking a glass of *lemonade* the impending attack is warded off. The free use of this beverage or of lemon-juice has often prevented, and in some instances seems to have cured old and inveterate headaches. It is an agreeable remedy and well worth a trial.

## VERTIGO OR GIDDINESS.

This affection may arise from a variety of causes, and so be cured by a variety of remedies. It may be a transient condition, or become chronic and comparatively permanent. It often arises from plethoric or full habit; from overloading the digestive organs, or from debilitating discharges, or from the use of narcotics.

TREATMENT.—When connected with full habit, red face, sparks before the eyes, etc., the Specific No. ONE is the remedy. If there is indigestion or overloaded stomach, take Specific No. TEN. If there have been debilitating discharges, such as diarrhœa, leucorrhœa, the No. TWENTY-FOUR will cure, or in some cases the No. TWENTY-EIGHT. Chronic vertigo, referable to no immediate producing cause, requires the Specific No. THIRTY-FIVE; dose, two pellets two or three times per day.

## APOPLEXY.

What is termed a fit of apoplexy, is a sudden loss of consciousness and motion, the patient sinking down as if dead, though the respiration and action of the heart continue in a somewhat irregular manner. It is different from spasm, the hands are not clenched or extremities rigid, but apparently dead and without motion. It is occasioned by an effusion of blood or of serum upon the brain, or from so intense a degree of congestion, as to paralyze the action of this organ. It is more important to know and arrest the premonitory symptoms, as after the attack has become fully developed, but comparatively little can be done by way of treatment. The subjects are mostly stout, plethoric people, of full habit and short necks, and it is more common in certain families having such physical conformation. The symptoms which point to an attack, are these: Great disposition to sleep; feeling of heaviness; dimness of sight; buzzing in the ears; hardness of hearing; heavy, deep sleep and loud snoring; yawning and fatigue after slight exertion; vertigo or giddiness; irritable disposition; loss of memory; forgetfulness of words or things; double or very acute vision; difficulty of swallowing; numbness, torpor or pricking sensation in the extremities; rush of blood to the head, with beating of the temporal arteries; red face and quick, hard, tense pulse. These symptoms are indicative of severe congestion of blood to the head, and unless arrested, may result in an effusion or fit of apoplexy.

TREATMENT.—This condition requires, first the use of the Specific No. ONE, if the symptoms are at all urgent; give two pellets every one or two hours until the oppression and sense of fulness is somewhat relieved, and in some cases this Specific will alone be sufficient for the time. Then commence and give the Specifics No. THIRTY-FIVE and No. TEN four times per day, two pellets at a time in alternation, as shown on page 52, until entirely relieved. Then to prevent a return, the No. THIRTY-FIVE should be taken each morning, and the No. TEN each night for some weeks, two pellets at a dose.

When a person falls down in a fit of apoplexy, which may be known from drunkenness by the absence of the smell of liquor in the breath, and from epilepsy by the absence of spasm in any part of the system, cold applications should at once be made to the head, and the feet should be immersed to the knees, if possible, in quite warm water, and the Specifics Nos. ONE and THIRTY-FIVE given dissolved in a few drops of water, at intervals of every half hour alternately, until animation is restored, and then at longer intervals as the patient improves. Afterwards, the Specifics Nos. TEN and THIRTY-FIVE may be continued to prevent a recurrence of the attack.

## CONGESTION, OR RUSH OF BLOOD TO THE HEAD.

Persons of full habit, and who lead a sedentary life, are subject to what is termed a rush of blood to the head. It is brought on or excited by intense or long-continued mental application, want of exercise, and often by too free indulgence in stimulating food, wine or alcoholic drinks.

The symptoms are: a sense of fulness in the head and neck; unusual beating or throbbing of the arteries throughout the body and head; heat, redness and bloating of the face, or sometimes paleness and puffing of the face; attacks of giddiness or vertigo, more after sleeping or sitting in a warm room, or from exposure to the sun; frequent headache, especially in the forehead, worse on coughing or stooping; buzzing or noise in the ears; oppressed breathing; dry, enlarged or reddish tongue; constipation; drowsiness by day and sleeplessness at night. These symptoms may come and go with the causes which excite them, or become a more or less permanent condition.

TREATMENT.—If the symptoms are urgent, dissolve eight or ten pellets of Specific No. ONE in six spoonfuls of water, of which take a spoonful every one or two hours until relieved; then, each morning, take two pellets of Specific No. THIRTY-FIVE, and each night two pellets of No. TEN, until every trace of the affection has disappeared.

## INFLAMMATION OF THE BRAIN—PHRENITIS ENCEPHALITIS.

The manifestations of this disease are varied very much by the age, sex and temperament of the patient, the location of the affection, and the causes which have produced it. Children, from the greater delicacy and relatively greater size of the organ, are far more liable to it than adults, and from greater delicacy of nervous organization, women are perhaps more so than men.

When the coverings or tissues of the brain are affected, the pain is more intense, and the symptoms more violent than when the substance of the organ is the seat of the disease; while in the latter case, the symptoms of dullness, coma and tendency to paralysis are more prominent.

CAUSES.—Whatever tends to overtask and excite this organ, is liable to induce the disease, such as extremes of heat or cold; abuse of ardent spirits; intense mental emotions; excesses of all kinds, or concussions of the brain; and in children especially, falls or blows upon the head, and overtaxing their faculties. And it may also be the result of repelled eruptions, or a metastasis of disease from some other organ.

The symptoms, which usually precede the attack for some days, are those indicating congestion of the blood to the head; sense of weight, fulness and pressure in the head; occasional darting or shooting pains; ringing in the ears and feverish symptoms. Farther on, the giddiness and sense of weight in the head are increased; pulse quickened, with some heat, restlessness and tossing at night; the mind becomes irritable, the patient peevish and annoyed at trifles; and there may be stupefaction and drowsiness, and muttering delirium or great excitability. The patient may be wild and frenzied at the slightest light or noise, with attempts to jump out of bed or run away; the eyes may be wild and bloodshot or turned up and distressed at the slightest approach of light. The fever varies according to the seat of the disease and the excitability of the patient; and the pulse varies from time to time, at one time quick or irregular, at another full or even slow. A very quick or very slow pulse indicates danger. Sometimes there is stupor or incontrollable vomiting; as the stupor increases convulsions commence, and the case sooner or later ends fatally.

In children, as only the objective symptoms can be known, it is of more importance to recognize them early. They are observed to manifest a heaviness of the head, by holding it backward when walking; frequently to hold the hand to the head from pain; to fall easily when walking or running; to dread the light, and to be easily annoyed or violently out of temper at trifles; or to have spells of vomiting and constipation, and to be drowsy or very wakeful, with startings during sleep.

As the case is more developed, the child bores with its head into the pillow; wants to lie down again when raised, and screams when the light shines in its face, or from any noise; or there is heavy, deep sleep, with great heat in the head; swelling and redness of the face; violent throbbing of the arteries of the neck, or great agitation and tossing about, especially at night; the eyes may be red and sparkling, convulsed or fixed, with dilated or very much contracted pupils.

TREATMENT.—The Specifics Nos. ONE and THIRTY-FIVE are our main reliance, and they should be given, dissolved in water, at intervals of every hour, or two hours, according to the urgency of the case. Dissolve twelve pellets of each of these Specifics in six large spoonfuls of water, separately, and give to adults a table, and to children a teaspoonful alternately from the two, at the intervals above mentioned, and so continue until the case is relieved.

Wet cloths may be applied with advantage to the head, and the feet from time to time bathed in quite warm water, if the condition of the patient admits it.

## DROPSY OF THE BRAIN—HYDROCEPHALUS.

This affection is not uncommon among small children, and sometimes even adults. It may come on as the sequel of scarlatina, inflammation or other acute disease of the brain, or in consequence of falls or blows upon the head, or be excited from the long-continued irritation of teething; or it may arise as an independent or idiopathic disease in peculiar subjects. Scrofulous children with large heads and precocious intellects, whose fontanel remains a long time open, are peculiarly liable to it. In some cases it comes on so insidiously that the premonitory symptoms escape attention altogether, while in others the impending disease is indicated by these symptoms: Hot skin, quick pulse, especially at night; the child is peevish and dislikes to be raised up when lying down, and sometimes has fits of screaming, redness of the face and eyes, and even at times squinting, convulsions or stupor.

When the disease comes on in the more insidious form, the earlier indications are: languor and easy fatigue on the slightest exertion; aversion to movement; tottering gait, and great liability to fall; dislike of movement; indications of pain in the back of the head and neck; the head is hot; eyes look inflamed; pupils contracted; the stomach is drawn in and very irritable; easily vomiting when the patient sits or is raised upright; scanty urine and constipated bowels.

At a more advanced stage the child loses all sense of pain; lies quiet unless disturbed; drowsiness or stupor increases; the head sinks or bores into the pillow; the eyes half closed; pupils dilated or immovable, or sometimes drawn to one side or attended with double vision; the vomiting becomes less or ceases, and the child may eat, but emaciation progresses rapidly. Following these symptoms, convulsions more or less violent come on; constant moaning and entire loss of consciousness; the eyes are dim, glazed and turned upward; pulse quick; the upper and lower extremities relaxed; the abdomen drawn up and breathing irregular, and the scene may terminate in a very violent convulsion.

TREATMENT.—So soon as any symptoms pointing to dropsy, or even irritation of the brain are manifested, the Specifics Nos. ONE and THIRTY-FIVE should be called into use, and two pellets be given alternately from these two Specifics, at intervals of two hours, until the danger has been averted.

Should the symptoms have become more decided, it will be best to dissolve twelve pellets from the Nos. ONE and THIRTY-FIVE, in as many teaspoonfuls of water, and from these two give alternately, every hour a spoonful until the desired relief is obtained.

Benefit will be derived from frequently bathing the feet in quite warm water, and afterwards wrapping them in warm flannels, and applying cloths wrung out of cold or ice water to the head. A bag of pounded ice applied to the head, is often very serviceable; and these measures should be continued perseveringly to the desired end. In extreme cases, the alternate use of the Nos. ONE and TWENTY-FIVE, given as above, is advisable; but, in general, the first mentioned remedies will prove sufficient.

## CHRONIC DROPSY OF THE BRAIN.

This form of the disease generally comes on insidiously, though it may be the result of the acute attack. The head of the child gradually enlarges, while the face retains its natural size; and in quite young children the bones of the cranium may separate, and the presence of fluid even be detected from its fluctuations. Emaciation, languor and lassitude are among the earlier symptoms, and gradually one or more of the senses become impaired or destroyed as the disease progresses. In some cases, the intellect is preserved for a considerable period. The head may attain such size that the patient cannot support it, and the attempt may be attended with giddiness, heat and pain in the head, or even vomiting; general or partial convulsions are liable to set in, sometimes resulting in permanent rigidity of the limbs, or only affecting certain muscles. In some cases, the child may live on for years, with entire loss of some of the senses, as for instance the sight, the general condition being otherwise, of tolerable health. The fatal termination is generally preceded by drowsiness, convulsions and general relaxation of the limbs; oftentimes the more immediate cause of death may be from some acute, inflammatory affection, consumption or ulceration of the bowels.

TREATMENT.—But little can be hoped for in the more confined cases of this disease. The Specifics No. THIRTY-FIVE and No. TWENTY-FIVE, may be given two or three times per day as palliatives, in alternation, but a cure can scarcely be expected unless in the earlier stages.

## CONVULSIONS; SPASMS, OR FITS.

Convulsions are very justly dreaded among children, not only because there is some danger attending them, but from their suddenness, and the evident distress and suffering of the patient. Their danger depends much upon the cause which has produced them. In some families the children have fits, as they are called, from very slight causes, and in such cases their appearance need not excite great alarm. Convulsions are dangerous when they set in after a fall, blow or injury upon the head, or after long continued disease of the brain, or after dropsy of the brain has set in; such are very frequently fatal precursors. They are of less consequence when they come on as the result of difficult teething, excessive pain, anger, earache, etc. Often in these cases, the patient is better after the convulsion has passed over. Not unfrequently a severe case of small-pox, scarlatina or measles is ushered in by an attack of convulsions. Though such cases are severe, they not unfrequently terminate favorably. If spasms appear towards the end of acute eruptive diseases, they are symptoms indicating a dangerous, if not fatal transition to the brain. The most common and among the most dangerous convulsions in children, are those arising from having eaten indigestible substances, such as raisins, oranges, dried-apples, nuts, green fruit, and similar indigestible articles, as the fit here depends upon the presence of the injurious substances, which it may be difficult to neutralize or dispose of. Yet even in these, the proper means will, in most cases, prove effectual.

The phenomenon of convulsion is well known. They often commence with holding back of the head; straightening out of the arms and legs; holding the breath; tightly clenching the hands; twitching of the muscles of the face; frothing at the mouth; involuntary evacuations, etc., after which the patient sinks into a deep sleep, lasting one or two hours.

Treatment.—When children are observed to have some degree of fever or heat of the head, and to twitch, or suddenly start on going to sleep, or attempting to do so, there is danger of convulsions, and the Specific No. One should be given, two pellets dry in the mouth, and repeated hourly until the surface becomes cool, and quiet sleep is produced. When a convulsion has come on, the first thing is to get the child's feet into warm water as high as the knees, if possible, which may be continued for five or ten minutes, and apply cold water by means of cloths wrung out of cold or even ice water to the head. Should the spasm not pass off from these applications, a small stream of cold water may be poured upon the head for a few minutes continuously, and the bath may be general; but these measures rarely will be required. Give also upon the tongue, two pellets of Specific No. THIRTY-THREE, and afterwards repeat it every hour in water. The child, after coming out of the bath, should be wrapped in warm flannels, with head quite high. Should there be fever, give the Specific No. ONE, the intermediate half hour between the portions of No. THIRTY-THREE, until the fever abates. This will be the appropriate treatment, should you have reason to suspect the invasion of small-pox or scarlatina as the cause of the disease.

If the convulsion has been caused by eating indigestible substances, in addition to the baths, lose no time in giving an *injection* of *tepid water*, in which a spoonful of salt has been dissolved, and repeat it if needful until full and free evacuations occur, giving the Specifics No. THIRTY-THREE and No. TEN, alternately every hour.

If irritation from teething has been the exciting cause, the Specific No. THREE should be given alternately with No. THIRTY-THREE, at intervals of an hour, and until the immediate danger is passed, and then the treatment continued as directed for teething.

## EPILEPSY.

This disease is characterized by convulsions, returning at intervals, attended with loss of consciousness and generally falling down with cries; foaming at the mouth, and with thumbs fixed beneath the fingers of the convulsed fist.

The fit is often unattended by any noticeable premonitory symptoms, but in some cases is preceded by pain in the head; sparks before the eyes; tingling in the ears; palpitations; languor, and a peculiar feeling beginning in some remote part of the system, such as the toes, fingers or abdomen, and rising towards the heart or head, with which consciousness disappears. The patient falls often with a scream; the arms and legs become convulsed; the hands clenched; body bent backward, forward or to either side; the jaws are set; respiration suspended or in sobs; the face drawn or violently convulsed; the eyeballs upturned; foam, often bloody from biting the tongue, issues from the mouth, and generally involuntary evacuations take place. Gradually, after a few moments, the spasms remit, the muscles become relaxed, respiration is restored, and the patient sinks into a deep sleep, from which he awakes quite recovered.

The paroxysm may soon return again if the occasioning cause is still in action, but generally in chronic cases, at intervals varying from a few days to several weeks. Sometimes patients have several fits in succession, and then escape them for several weeks.

But few persons die in a fit, but they may be repeated so frequently as to induce a comatose state, from which the patient sinks. Long continuance of the disease rarely fails to affect the mental faculties, and idiocy, more or less complete is a very common result.

When the disease commences before the age of puberty, it is more amenable to the proper treatment than afterwards, though in the latter cases, we are able to do very much by way of mitigating and prolonging the intervals between the convulsions, and in many instances to effect a cure.

Treatment.—During a fit the patient should receive only such attention as will prevent injury from the convulsive movements. Remove or loosen the cravat from the neck, and stays from the body, and prevent the limbs from being bruised, and if the tongue is liable to be lacerated, something may be inserted between the teeth to prevent it. If the breathing is arrested for a dangerous period, by spasm of the respiratory muscles, cold water may be sprinkled in the face to return it. The body should be placed in a horizontal position and the head elevated. After the patient has come out of the fit, he should be allowed to rest quietly an hour or two until he awakes.

The medical treatment consists in giving two pellets of the Specific No. THIRTY-FIVE each morning, and the same of No. THIRTY-THREE each evening, which should be continued for several weeks or even months.

Persons subject to fits should be very particular in regard to diet. Eat only plain food, easy of digestion, and in great moderation. Where there is a full habit and tendency to congestion, stimulants should be entirely avoided.

## ST. VITUS' DANCE—CHOREA.

This disease mostly effects children of nervous temperament, between the ages of five and fifteen years, and is characterized by strange and unusual movements and jerkings of the limbs, or of single muscles.

Generally, for some months previous to the full manifestation of the disease, the child is troubled with constipation, oppression of the stomach or chest, vertigo or headache, occasional flushes of fever at night, palpitation of the heart, nervousness and irritability of temper. Involuntary motions generally commence with grimaces or slight motions or drawings of the face; these gradually become more decided and extend by degrees to the extremities, arms, hands or legs, and even to the entire body. When the limbs are affected, the gait becomes difficult, awkward or unsteady. The arms fail to obey the will, and then involuntary motions or gestures, and if the tongue becomes involved, the act of deglutition is impeded, and the speech becomes stammering or difficult. The involuntary motions are constant during the waking hours, and some cases are attended with difficult respiration, pain in the limbs, frequent micturition, confusion of ideas, and loss of memory.

It is usually unattended with danger, and often subsides at the age of puberty, but it may also become permanent, and be attended by perversion or permanent weakening of the mental powers. It has frequently been caused by repelled eruptions, such as tetter, scald-head or itch, also from depressing emotions, fear, terror, masturbation, or the irritation of worms. Overtaxing the mental powers at school, and too long school hours is a most frequent cause.

TREATMENT.—The Specifics Nos. THIRTY-THREE and THIRTY-FIVE will usually be found effectual. Give two pellets of the latter at night, and the same from the former each morning, and with the removal of the exciting cause, the health will gradually be restored.

## TETANUS—LOCKJAW.

This disease is usually the result of some injury or wound, sometimes apparently trivial, such as lacerating the hand, or wounding the foot by a nail, or it may come on after surgical operations by which a nerve is compromised, or it may in rare cases be the result of a cold. The injury to the nerve or tendon acting upon a peculiar nervous condition, is the supposed cause of the general spasm termed lockjaw.

In some cases it commences suddenly and with great violence, but it more frequently begins by degrees; commencing with slight stiffness in the back part of the neck, and an uneasy sensation at the root of the tongue, which gradually increases, attended with difficulty of swallowing, oppressive tightness of the chest, and pain under the breast bone extending to the back; the countenance becomes pale; pulse small; urine high colored, and bowels constipated. The lower jaw becomes immovable and tightly clenched, so that at times the slightest particle cannot be inserted between them, hence the name lockjaw arises. In some cases the spasm is confined to the jaws, but in others they extend with increasing frequency to the arms, legs, and even the entire body, bending it backwards, forwards, or to either side. In the worst cases, the tetanus becomes general, the eyes fixed and immovable, and the countenance distorted with an expression of anguish; the body and limbs fixed, or with frequently occuring spasms, drawn in different directions, until nature becomes exhausted and succumbs at about the fourth day in a continued general spasm. Sometimes, during the remission of spasms, they are renewed by the patient moving, speaking, or taking food or drink.

TREATMENT.—After wounds or injuries, especially laceration or punctures with rough instruments, spikes, nails, etc., in the hands or feet, great care should be taken to subdue the irritation and inflammatory action, and to have the wound heal kindly. To this end, dress the wound with WITCH HAZEL, and keep the dressing moist with it for some days; avoid working with it, or irritating it, and especially avoid taking cold. The wound will thus heal up kindly, with no evil result.

Should symptoms of lockjaw appear, give at once the Specifics No. THIRTY-THREE and No. THIRTY-FIVE in alternation every hour, a dose of two pellets dissolved in water, and continue these without intermission until the spasm has entirely ceased.

When, from the constant clenching of the jaws, it is difficult to administer the medicine in the common method, let the pellets be dissolved in only a few drops of water, and be drawn in with the breath, or even be put in between the lips.

Cases of extreme tetanus have been cured by placing the patient sitting in a tub or bath, and pouring a stream of *cold water* continuously over the head and shoulders and down the spine, until *violent, cold shivering* is produced, when the patient will be found to be relaxed, and should be wiped dry, wrapped in blankets and put to bed. The operation will rarely have to be repeated, and is a very simple remedy and may be tried when others fail.

## NEURALGIA—PAIN IN A NERVE.

This is a comparatively modern and very common as well as painful affection. As the name indicates, it is simply pain in a nerve, and hence it may exist in any part of the body. It is very common in the face, (prosopalgy,) the pain frequently extending from just before the ear, along under and up over the eye, or it may descend along the face and lower jaw of that side to the center of the face; or it may extend to and along the root of the teeth. The pain is violent, sharp or rending, tearing or lancinating, often coming with paroxysm of increase and remission, and often very regularly better or worse at certain periods of the day or night. Sometimes the entire head or side are involved, and the patient can scarcely describe his symptoms. The pain is not increased, but generally diminished by pressure on the affected part, in distinction from pain of an inflammatory or rheumatic character, where pressure increases the pain.

TREATMENT.—The Specific No. EIGHT will usually be found sufficient, and may be given in portions of two pellets dry on the tongue, and repeated every one or two hours, according to circumstances.

In cases of chronic neuralgia, the Specific No. THIRTY-

FIVE may be given in alternation with the No. EIGHT, and two pellets of each be given twice per day, making four or six doses in all.

Sometimes, in very violent attacks, attended with fever, red face, or heat of the head, the Specific No. ONE may be efficient, dissolved in water, twelve pellets in six spoonfuls, and a spoonful given every hour. The use of the above named remedies will usually be found effective, even in the severest cases.

## TOOTHACHE.

*Toothache* is an affection so well known as to require no description. The pain is usually found in connection with decayed teeth, but sometimes also in sound ones. When badly decayed teeth begin to ache, it may be best to have them extracted. Yet, even here, the proper Specific treatment will often entirely allay the pain, and the teeth may do good service for many years afterwards. But when pain affects sound teeth, we should rarely submit to have them taken out, until we have exhausted every means to relieve them without this alternative. A most insane practice it is, whenever we have a toothache, which may be occasioned from a cold and will hence soon pass off, or from a bad state of the stomach, or by fever, or from mental and physical excitement, or from drinking coffee, or pregnancy—all transient conditions—to rush to the doctor or dentist and lose a tooth—a loss which can never be repaired. Under such circumstances, if we will exercise a little patience, a little discretion and judgment, we may allay the pain, remove the exciting cause and save the tooth as well as the suffering of its extraction.

TREATMENT.—Take first, two pills of the Specific No. EIGHT and repeat them every hour if needful. If not relieved, dissolve six or eight of the pills in a glass half full of water; also prepare the Specific No. ONE in the same manner and take them alternately every hour, or every two hours, until relieved. Sometimes the Specific No. FIFTEEN is very efficient, especially in rheumatic subjects, or when the pains appear to have a rheumatic origin, and in other cases the Dyspepsia pills are equally so.

When the toothache does not seem to yield, and especially in children who are fretful and impatient, relief may be obtained by bathing the face on the affected side freely with WITCH HAZEL, and holding some of it in the mouth on that side. If the tooth is hollow, wet a little pledget of lint with the same, and press it into the cavity of the tooth. Even better than bathing the face in the same, is wetting a thin cloth or handkerchief with the same, and wrapping it over the affected parts of the face or jaw with a handkerchief.

It is a bad practice in toothache, to hold camphor spirits or other stimulants in the mouth, or to apply creosote, laudanum, oil of cloves, etc., to the teeth. These more frequently irritate than relieve—excite and irritate the entire mouth and gums, and do more harm than good. Let the diet be light if the stomach is deranged; if there is a cold, cure that, and you will soon find relief, and save your teeth. If relieved an hour or so after taking the remedies, take no more; if it returns, try another dose, and even repeat it after an hour or two. Often a single portion will cure a severe case.

## SWELLED FACE.

Not unfrequently, and often as the sequel of toothache, the face, more especially on one side, becomes swelled or puffed out sometimes to an extreme degree. The entire tissue of the cheek and sometimes the face, becomes thickened and swelled so as to distort the countenance, and render deglutition or even opening the mouth difficult or painful.

The swelling may be red and hot with heat, and some degree of fever or even erysipelatious, or it may be pale or hard.

It is not a very dangerous affair, but sufficiently disagreeable and unpleasant to require attention, and more especially so when it assumes the graver forms.

TREATMENT.—If the swelling is red or hot, or both, with some fever, the Specific No. ONE is the remedy, and may be given in doses of two pellets dissolved in water, and repeated every two hours. If the swelling is firm or hard, alternate No. FIFTEEN in like manner with No. ONE; or if the toothache has been cured by the No. EIGHT, its continuous use will also cure the swelling of the face.

In painful swelling of the face, the application of a cloth wet in WITCH HAZEL will relieve both the pain and swelling.

# DISEASES OF THE EYES.

The eye, from its importance and the delicate nature of its structure, ought to claim our most careful attention when it is the subject of disease. We should, at all times, be careful not to apply salves, ointments or irritating washes, but to treat this organ with the utmost caution and tenderness, only applying those substances herein recommended, trusting mainly to the action of the remedies given internally. Nor should we be too hasty in intrusting them to the care of ignorant or ill-advised pretenders.

It should be recollected that in all cases of diseased or sore eyes, though the affection seems to be local, yet the whole system is more or less in sympathy with it; and often the local affection is only the expression of a general morbid condition of the system. Thus it is that scrofula, gout, rhematism, catarrh, or syphilis, may each locate themselves upon the eyes, producing their peculiar forms of inflammation or disease, and hence in the process of cure, those remedies appropriate to these conditions should be employed in connection with those for the local disease.

## ACUTE OPHTHALMY—INFLAMMATION OF THE EYE.

The attack often commences with a feeling as if sand or dust had got into the eye, the eyeball and inside of the lid become reddened, and the vessels distributed over the eye injected, carrying red blood. The eyes become irritated, intolerant of light and painful, with flow of hot, scalding tears.

In some forms, where the inflammation runs high or continues long, ulcers or small specks are apt to form upon the cornea or ball of the eye.

TREATMENT.—For the first twenty-four or forty-eight hours, give the Specifics No. ONE and No. EIGHTEEN in alternation, a dose every three hours. Prepare the medicine by dissolving six pellets of each in six spoonfuls of water in separate glasses, and administer from the two in alternation. After two days omit the Specific No. ONE, and instead use the Specific No. THIRTY-FIVE in like manner, in alternation with No. EIGHTEEN. As the inflammation subsides and the eye improves, the medicine may be taken less frequently, and, the medicine may be taken dry, two pellets at a time, instead of in fluid form.

Let the eye be shaded from light if it is oppressive, and avoid reading, writing or taxing the eye in any manner, and live on very light, easily digested food.

For an application, use WITCH HAZEL diluted with an equal quantity of pure, soft water, and with this bathe the eye, and at night wet a fine linen rag with it and lay over the eye, renewing from time to time as it gets hot or dry. If the same cannot be procured, dissolve ten pellets of Specific No. EIGHTEEN in half a teacupful of soft water, and use in like manner.

In cases where scrofula or rheumatism are clearly connected with the disease as a cause, it may be advisable, should the cure linger, to alternate the Specifics for those diseases, No. TWENTY-THREE or No. FIFTEEN, with that for ophthalmy, No. EIGHTEEN.

## CHRONIC OPHTHALMY.

Inflammations of the eyes are often met with of many months, and even years standing. They are sometimes better for a season and then worse again, and generally have their origin in some constitutional taint or dyscrasia of the system, such as gout or scrofula, or they may arise from the virus of syphilis or gonorrhœa. The eyeball is generally reddened, vessel injected, lids thickened, red and swelled; intolerance of light, and discharge of thick or purulent matter, or of hot, scalding water, when the irritation has been kindled up afresh. Ulcers, or the remains of old ulcers, are not unfrequently met with.

Treatment.—These old cases, which are often met with in bad, unhealthy or neglected subjects, only require care and patience in their treatment. Under good management, wonders can be effected in restoring these organs to sight and usefulness. Give at first, the Specifics No. Eighteen and No. Thirty-five, two pills at a time and four times per day in alternation. Continue this course a week or two weeks, or as long as the eyes continue to improve. If, after a time, the secretion is thick, gummy or abundant, omit the No. Thirty-five and use the No. Twenty-three instead, and so continue for one or two weeks, returning again to the former medicine to complete the cure.

The diet may be more generous than in acute ophthalmy, but still should be free from stimulants of any kind.

## INFLAMMATION OF THE EYELIDS.

Not unfrequently the eyelid becomes inflamed, red, swelled and painful, especially along the margin of the lid, while the eyeball seems but slightly affected. In some cases the frequent recurrence or persistence of this affection, causes the thickening of the margin of the lid, and the permanent loss of the eyelashes.

Treatment.—The Specifics Nos. Eleven and Eighteen are the appropriate medicines, and may be administered two or four times per day according to the urgency of the case, as directed for acute ophthalmy.

## STY.

This is a small, hard, generally inflamed tumor, seated on the margin of the lid, commencing as a small, painful lump, becoming inflamed, swelled, red, and finally softening. In some cases a tumor like a small wen appears in the same locality, and remains without suppurating or discharging.

TREATMENT.—It will be speedily removed by the use of the Specifics Nos. EIGHTEEN and ELEVEN in alternation. A dose of two pellets may be given every two or three hours at first, then morning and night is sufficient. Small, indolent tumors or wens may require the use of Nos. EIGHTEEN and THIRTY-FIVE, given two pellets night and morning.

## BLOOD-SHOT EYES.

Sometimes from severe or violent coughing, blows, falls, retching, vomiting or crying, the eye or a portion of it becomes suffused with blood, or bloodshot as it is termed. It generally passes off itself by being absorbed when the occasioning cause has ceased to act. A few doses of Specific No. THIRTY-FIVE, given two or three times per day, will hasten the removal of the extravasation. Frequent bathing with WITCH HAZEL may also hasten the absorption.

## WATERY, WEEPING EYES.

When this is the result of the closure or obliteration of the tear-duct, medicine will not avail. But when it arises from weakness or over sensibility of the organ, or a partial closure of the duct from inflammatory thickening of the surrounding tissue, or from the secretion itself being thickened, it is quite within the reach of medical treatment.

Administer in such cases the Specific No. EIGHTEEN, two pellets two or three times per day. If a catarrhal condition at the same time exists, interpose an occasional dose of two pellets of Specific No. NINETEEN.

## SQUINTING—STRABISMUS.

This affection, in its more serious form, can only be reached by a surgical operation. But in some cases of comparatively recent origin in young children, it may be corrected by the use of the Specific No. THIRTY-FIVE, two pellets given morning and night.

## WEAK, OR FAILING SIGHT.

In many cases, the sight fails or becomes obscured or feeble before that period of life when it may naturally be expected. Sometimes, there is a mist or gauze before the eyes, or there are black points, spots or clouds hovering before the sight; or the eyes become dim, watery, or the sight misty on endeavoring to sew, read or use fine print. These conditions indicate weakness of these organs, or a morbid condition of them, and it may be but the reflection of the general condition of the system.

TREATMENT.—Take two pellets of the Specific No. THIRTY-FIVE each morning, and the same of No. EIGHTEEN every night on retiring. Also, frequently bathe the eyes with cold water, avoid fatiguing or straining the eyes with fine work, reading fine print, or any long continued effort of the eyes, and also the use of glasses, which fatigue or weary the eyes. In all cases, avoid fatiguing or taxing the eyes when the body is weak and enfeebled from sickness.

# AFFECTIONS OF THE EARS AND HEARING.

## EARACHE—INFLAMMATION OF THE EAR.

Earache may have a neuralgic or rheumatic origin, or even from toothache, and is very common in children. It is often brought on from exposure to cold, rough or damp weather. The pain is usually severe, sharp, lancinating or beating, extending deep into the ear, causing great suffering. In very young children it occasions great uneasiness, cries, and rolling of the head. When the ear becomes inflamed, the brain may become implicated from the extension of the disease, and delirium or convulsions with vomiting and cold extremities may be the result. In many instances, when young children have been crying, fretful and peevish for several days, a discharge from the ear first informs the nurse that an inflammation of the ear has been the cause of all the suffering.

TREATMENT.—The principal Specifics are the No. ONE and No. TWENTY-TWO. Give first the No. ONE, two pellets every hour, either dry or dissolved in a spoonful of water, and for simple otalgia or earache it will suffice. If the case is complicated with inflammation, very severe pains or redness of the external ear, or of the passage, as is not unfrequently the case, give Specific No. ELEVEN, two pellets every hour, either alone or in alternation with No. ONE until the disease has yielded, and for any remaining swelling or discharge give the No. TWENTY-TWO, two pellets four times per day.

In severe cases, a little cotton-wool wet with WITCH HAZEL and placed gently in the ear, affords prompt relief, and may at any time be resorted to.

## DISCHARGE FROM THE EAR—OTORRHŒA.

Discharges from the ear frequently remain for a time after the acute affection has disappeared. But it is also frequently the result of scarlet fever, measles, or of some scrofulous development. Repeated attacks of earache are quite sure to result in long continued discharges from the ear, with its concomitant results, noises in the head, and hardness of hearing. The discharge is sometimes fetid, offensive, thick, green, cream-like, varying in consistence, quantity and character.

TREATMENT.—The successful treatment of old, long standing otorrhœa, requires some time and patience. It cannot be done at once, but fortunately can be accomplished, and the hearing of the organ generally preserved. The Specific No. TWENTY-TWO, two pellets three times per day, will generally accomplish the desired result. Sometimes the occasional interposition of a dose of Specific No. THIRTY-FIVE accelerates the cure.

## DIFFICULT HEARING; NOISES IN THE HEAD.

These two affections may properly be considered in connection. Buzzing, roaring, whizzing, and other noises in the head are often the incipient stage of deafness, and the noise must of necessity impair the hearing. Noises in the head may result from a cold or some obstruction, or be the consequence of a running or discharge from the ear. Hardness of hearing may result from any of the cases heretofore named, or from dryness of the ear, insufficient secretion of the cerumen or ear-wax, or various morbid conditions of the internal ear. The ear should be examined and any accumulations of wax carefully removed. If the ear or wax is dry or hard, drop in a drop or two of pure glycerine night and morning until the wax is softened, or the dryness removed.

Syringing the ear as it is often done results in more harm than good. The less water or soap in the ear the better, aside from mere purposes of cleanliness. Recent cases are often cured, while the old and long-standing are not unfrequently obstinate, or, if the bone is involved, intractable.

TREATMENT.—The Specific No. TWENTY-TWO is in general the remedy, and may be administered either for noises in the head or hardness of hearing, two pellets night and morning. If after eight or ten days there is no decided improvement, use the Specific No. THIRTY-FIVE, in like manner for eight days, and again return to the first prescription, and so continue for weeks, or months if necessary, using one medicine *for eight days at a time* and then resorting to the other.

## ACUTE CATARRH—INFLUENZA—GRIPPE.

An attack of acute catarrh is generally manifested by sneezing often repeated, followed by a sensation of irritation, itching or tingling, extending along the nasal passages to the head and throat, and often down along the larynx and bronchia into the lungs. To this there may be added coryza, tearfulness and weeping from the eyes and discharge of mucus from the nose at first, thin, acrid, irritating and gradually becoming more copious, thick, yellow, and sometimes offensive, as the disease subsides. To this is sometimes added sore throat, cough and irritation of the lungs.

Where many people are attacked during the same period with the above symptoms, which are, however, often widely modified, but always attended with a *degree of debility, prostration* and persistence of symptoms above what is warranted by the local irritation, it is usually denominated Grippe or Influenza.

TREATMENT.—The Specifics NOS. NINETEEN and SEVEN

are usually all that is required. Should there be considerable fever or heat of the surface, either at once or succeeding a chill, it will be best to commence with Specific No. ONE, and give of this every hour two pellets dissolved in water until the fever abates. Then give the Specific No. NINETEEN every two hours, two pellets alone; or, if there is some cough or bronchial irritation, alternate Specific No. SEVEN with it at the same intervals until the disease is subdued.

## CHRONIC CATARRH.

Chronic catarrh often may be said to be constitutional. In some families every member is affected with it more or less. From the first years of childhood, there is an excessive secretion from the nose and air passages. The disease is characterized by an excessive flow of mucus, more or less changed, from the lining membrane of the nose and its back passages, the frontal sinus and throat, and sometimes involving the bronchia and lungs. The discharge is varied in color, character and consistence. Often it is yellow, thick, abundant and offensive, or it may be drier, in plugs or crusts, obstructing the passages and only detached occasionally and with difficulty, accompanied with soreness or ulceration. Sometimes the membrane lining the passage is very red and painfully irritated from every inhalation of the air, and the discharge watery, thin and acrid; but the most common form is the profuse discharge of yellow, thick, offensive matter. Generally the sense of smell is impaired and sometimes quite lost, and not unfrequently the sense of hearing and taste are likewise more or less impaired. Though a chronic catarrh may continue many years and be very annoying and offensive, it is rarely fatal, and I think never terminates in consumption, whatever quacks may say about it. It is generally better in warm, dry weather, and worse in the spring and fall and in variable weather.

TREATMENT.—The Specific No. NINETEEN is the proper remedy, and may be given, two pellets at a time and from two to four times per day, according to the urgency of the case. Should there be bronchial irritation, cough or hoarseness, the Specific No. SEVEN may be used in alternation with No. NINETEEN to good advantage.

## FALL CATARRH—PEACH CATARRH—HAY ASTHMA.

This is a peculiar torm of catarrh, to which many persons, especially in the better walks of life, are subject, and which has received quite a variety of designations. It comes on at rarely varying periods, generally about the 20th of August, and having made its attack, is almost sure to return every year at about the same day. It continues with varying degrees of intensity until about the first of October or the first cold or frosty day, when it gradually abates. The attack commences with sneezing, commonly violent and repeated, to which there is soon added tearfulness and discharge of thin watery secretion from the nose, sometimes so abundant as to fall in drops or to soil a dozen or more handkerchiefs in a day. The eyes become watery, the lining membrane of the lids red and irritated, the lining membrane of the nose reddened and exceedingly irritated from the dust of traveling or the pollen of flowers. Gradually the irritation extends along the air passage, involving the bronchia, and paroxysms of asthma set in, worse at night, obliging the patient to sit bolstered up, and rendering a horizontal position for the time impossible. While the difficulty of breathing is so great, the discharge from the eyes and nose and the sneezing abates, but after two or three days the asthma passes off and the eyes and nose have it again. And so the disease wears on with varying degrees of severity from bad to worse, until time and the cooler days afford relief from this most disagreeable and annoying of physical visitations.

Numerous theories have been advanced as to the cause of this annual catarrh. It has been attributed to the down of peaches, the fragrance of roses, the dust of making hay, the pollen of flowers, etc. But whether any or all of these theories are correct, it seems clearly to be connected with an advanced stage, or possibly, an incipient decay of some forms of vegetation; for we find it cured for the time by a sea voyage, and patients suffering from it who domicile in those locations most removed from such influences are proportionately relieved. Thus, those who go to the Catskill Mountain House say they are sensibly benefited, and those at Fire Island, where scores of fashionable people, who flee from this visitant, are to be found every year, as certainly as the returning swallows, aver that they suffer only about one fourth as much as when on the main land.

Old school medicine has accomplished little or nothing toward relieving this class of patients, and the Homeopaths have not done much better, patients of the most distinguished physicians of all schools in our large cities being found in abundance at these places of refuge every year.

TREATMENT.—If the patient can sojourn for the time at any of the localities named, or can take a sea voyage, it is to be advised. The Specifics Nos. NINETEEN and TWENTY-ONE had best be taken—two pills, from one at night and the other in the morning, for some days before the expected attack, to ward it off if possible. When the attack comes on, commence at once with these two numbers and take two pills every two hours alternately either dry or dissolved in water, and continue this at longer intervals as the disease abates. When the eyes are much affected with redness, intolerance of light, and profuse tearfulness, suspend the No. NINETEEN and take instead No. EIGHTEEN, every two hours two pills, and so continue them until the irritation of the eyes are relieved.

Thus these three Specifics may be used, either alone or in alternation with each other during the course of the disease. You will thus relieve, shorten and wonderfully modify, if you do not entirely arrest, this most unpleasant, if not dangerous annual visitation.

# DISEASES OF THE AIR PASSAGES.

---

## HOARSENESS.

This affection is common, and generally the result of a cold or some irritation at the upper portion of the windpipe or larynx. It is sometimes deserving of serious attention, as it may indicate changes in the upper part of the larynx of a very grave character. It is also a symptom in croup, laryngitis, bronchitis and measles. Sometimes the voice is wholly lost, the patient being only able to speak in whispers ; at others, it is low, rough, hoarse or piping.

TREATMENT.—When the hoarseness is the result of a cold, bronchitis, or other disease, no particular attention need be paid to this particular symptom. It will disappear under the use of the Specifics given for the general disease. When it is idiopathic, or even the most prominent symptom, the Specific No. SEVEN, two pills every two or three hours, will soon restore the voice. In cases of chronic hoarseness or loss of voice, give two pellets of Specific No. SEVEN, three times per day, continuing the same until relief is obtained.

Clergymen, after speaking, or persons who, after singing, find the voice fatigued, hoarse, furzy, or the throat irritated, will find relief from taking of the Specific No. SEVEN, two pills at once, and the portion may be repeated at intervals of three hours, until the unpleasant sensation or hoarseness has disappeared.

## CROUP.

Croup is usually a disease of childhood, nevertheless there are some adults who are sometimes subject to it in a quite serious form. In children it is always a serious and sometimes a suddenly fatal disease, and hence it is important to be acquainted with its earlier symptoms in order to be able to arrest them. Children from fifteen months to five or seven years of age are most subject to it. Often it comes on suddenly at night, after the child has been exposed or out playing in a damp, cold or rough wind during the day. The child wakes out of sleep with a sudden hoarse, rough, barking cough, often like the barking of an old dog, and often even at first a hoarseness or difficulty in speaking, and a degree of anxiety with difficulty of breathing. In some cases there are frequent returns of this hoarse, rough, croupy cough, with little or no fever, or difficulty of breathing for some hours, or even a day or two; and the child runs about and is even at times playful until the full disease is ushered in. At others, there is high fever, quick pulse, red face, hoarse cough and difficult breathing from the first hour of the attack. As the disease progresses the fever increases, the cough returns in more frequent paroxysms, is more harsh, dry and tight, and the difficulty of breathing increases, (often by paroxysms,) becomes wheezing, with rustling of mucus, labored, and in the worst cases as if breathing through fine brazen pipes, and by degrees becomes loud and harsh, and may be heard all over the room or even the house. Towards the last the breathing becomes increasingly difficult, the voice fails, or is only heard in whispers, the head is thrown backward to facilitate respiration, the larynx rises and falls with every breath, and the child is bathed in perspiration from the suffering and effort. If the child improves, the breathing becomes easier, freer, and the rattling of mucus looser; the cough more loose and moist, and the voice more natural. If worse, the breathing is more difficult, finer-toned and tighter, the cough dryer, and voice failing.

Sudden attacks of croup are usually not so formidable, and sooner yield to proper treatment. But the worst cases of croup (angina membranacea) come on more insidiously. The child may be considered only slightly unwell for several days, *with little or no cough*, or a *mild, veiled cough*, but the *speech* is *changed* and is a *hoarse whispering* or is *entirely lost*, and in these cases the difficulty of breathing comes on very gradually, and may not be noticed except on careful observation, or when the child is making some effort. Such insidious cases are always dangerous and often fatal, and this symptom of *loss of voice or whispering voice in children* should always demand attention. It generally marks the deposition or formation of the false membrane, and requires only its continued deposition to become fatal.

TREATMENT.—For the hoarse, croupy cough that often precedes the croup, the Specific No. THIRTEEN will be sufficient, giving two pills every two or three hours, and keeping the child well housed and protected from the cold, and especially from exposure to rough, damp air. Where an attack comes on with hoarse cough and some difficulty of breathing, dissolve the Specifics Nos. ONE and THIRTEEN, six or eight pellets of each, in as many teaspoonfuls of water in separate glasses, and give the child a spoonful alternately every fifteen minutes, first from No. ONE, and next from No. THIRTEEN, and so on in alternation, if the case is urgent, with these two medicines, only prolonging the intervals between the medicines to half an hour or an hour, as the patient improves. After the fever abates and the cough becomes moist or assumes its natural tone, and the breathing is relieved and free perspiration established, the No. ONE may be discontinued and the No. THIRTEEN continued until the cure is completed.

It is quite useless and pernicious to give castor oil, hive syrup, epicac, or to rub over the chest oil, goose-grease, or similar substances, as is often done. Simply make the child comfortable, keep it well covered in bed or in the nurse's lap, and in a mildly warm room free from exposure or drafts of air, and give the Specifics as directed, and the vast majority of cases of croup will terminate favorably. Care should also be taken not to expose children to the cold or to let them go out too soon after an attack of croup. They should be kept well housed and protected until entirely recovered, to prevent a relapse.

## COUGH.

Cough is in general only a symptom of some other disease, such as catarrh, bronchitis, inflammation or congestion of the lungs, or the bronchia, or influenza, whooping-cough, etc.; and the cure of the cough will have to be effected by the cure of the disease upon which it depends. But in many cases the cough may be the principal, and perhaps the only indication of diseased action, and hence demand treatment of itself. Often it is the forerunner or first stage of some disease which is thus cured through the indications furnished by the cough. A suspicious cough, especially in persons of delicate health, or weak lungs, should never be permitted to continue from week to week, but should always excite our suspicion and demand the persistent use of the proper measures for its relief.

TREATMENT.—In general the Specific No. SEVEN will be sufficient. Give two pellets, dry or in water, four times per day, avoiding exposure to new irritation, and the desired end will generally soon be reached.

Should the cough, however, be harsh and dry, with some fever or pain in the chest or side, it is better to alternate the No. ONE with the No. SEVEN, giving a portion of two pellets every two hours alternately, until the cough is relieved.

*Violent spasmodic coughs*, approaching hooping-coughs, often require the use of Specific No. TWENTY, either alone or in alternation with No. SEVEN, given as directed above.

*Old chronic coughs*, of long standing, are often cured by the No. SEVEN and No. THIRTY-FIVE, in alternation, given two or four times per day, preferably before meals and on retiring at night. If the case is urgent, the medicine may be given, a portion every three hours.

## HOOPING COUGH.

This disease, like scarlet fever and measles, may be communicated from one child to another by means of the breath, expectoration, or even the exhalations from the persons affected, and rarely attacks the same individual the second time. It is more severe and dangerous in some seasons than at others, and though under Homeopathic treatment but few hooping cough patients are lost, yet it is often a troublesome disease, and not unfrequently, under bad management, or in severe cases, leaves serious after sufferings in its train. Under Specific treatment, it generally passes off as a mild and not tedious visitation.

It usually commences as a common cold, with cough, some fever, hoarseness, sneezing, or running from the nose, and this catarrhal stage may continue for eight, ten or fourteen days, before the true character of the disease is manifested. But the cough, if carefully noticed, has from the first a more spasmodic or convulsive character than a common cold, and by degrees its true form is developed, namely: *severe shocks of cough, following each other in rapid succession, succeeded by a deep inhalation or hoop.* Often there are two paroxysms following in succession, succeeded by an interval of half an hour or more, according to the intensity of the irritation. Frequently, food is vomited by the convulsive effort of the coughing, and sneezing, bleeding from the nose, blood-shot eyes, or even convulsions in extreme cases, are not uncommon.

The disease gradually grows worse until at each paroxysm of cough there is a free expectoration of tough, viscid mucus, when, having reached its acme, it as gradually declines to the end; unless, indeed, a new cold is taken, or a fresh irritation set up, when the disease relapses and a part of the ground is gone over again. Uncontrolled by treatment, the disease often lasts twelve weeks, or even a longer period, while treated by our simple method, one half or fourth of that period is sufficient for a cure.

TREATMENT.—If the disease is prevailing, or children have been exposed to this disease, and you do not wish them to have it, give the Specific No. TWENTY, two pellets three times per day, and you will generally prevent its access.

Should the disease have commenced as a common cold, with cough, fever, sneezing, or sore throat, give the Specific No. ONE and No. SEVEN for one or two days, two pellets at a time, every two hours in alternation, and after that omit the No. SEVEN, and instead give the No. TWENTY, in the same manner; and as soon as the feverish condition has subsided, omit the No. ONE and give only the No. TWENTY, two pellets four times per day, and so continue during the course of the disease.

If during the course of the disease the cough becomes frequent, tight, dry, and it loses the usual hooping sound, and with some fever, indicating the access of inflammation of the bronchia, or of the substance of the lung, at once return to the Specific No. ONE, and give ten pellets every hour in solution until the threatening symptoms have been warded off, and then go on again with No. TWENTY, either alone or in alternation with No. ONE.

Often by taking the disease at the commencement, you

will arrest its progress before its full development, and it will pass off in a week or two as a mere catarrhal cough, having never reached the hooping-cough form.

During the disease, the child should be carefully nursed and fed on light, easily digested diet, with but little or no meat, avoiding cake or rich, heavy food, pies or sweetmeats; but, on the contrary, giving an abundance of mucilaginous drinks, such as gum-water, rice-water, barley-water, Iceland moss, weak chicken or lamb broth, or weak black tea or chocolate.

Vaccination during hooping-cough usually causes the disease to run a very mild course, and if it has been omitted until this period, it may be well to have it then performed.

## ACUTE BRONCHITIS—COMMON COLD—BRONCHIAL IRRITATION.

These conditions have so many symptoms in common, and so frequently run into and overlap each other, that it is preferable to treat them in connection. Laymen would find it difficult to distinguish one from the other, nor would it be necessary in a practical point of view. A cold generally commences with a sensation of tingling, itching, irritation, or roughness along the lining membrane of the nose, and thence gradually extending backward along the air passage into the bronchia or lungs. There is often sneezing, sometimes repeated, and soon a discharge, at first of thin acrid, and then by degrees thicker, yellowish mucus from the nose, and cough, at first harsh, dry, violent, often accompanied with a sense of roughness or excoriation in the larynx and upper part of the chest, and as the disease progresses, raising of at first thin, and then more thick, or yellowish sputa. Sometimes the bronchia and chest are but little affected, and the disease expends itself upon the mucus membrane of the throat, nose and eyes, producing frequent sneezing, redness and irritation of the eyes, and profuse secretion of the acrid mucus from the eyes and nose. When the bronchia is particularly invaded, the cough is dry, harsh, painful and frequent, often inducing headache, together with more or less hoarseness, and sore throat if the upper part of wind-pipe (larynx) is involved. Fever to a greater or more limited extent is almost always present, and the disease presents all grades, from a sharp, well defined, acute bronchitis to a simple catarrhal irritation. As the disease declines, and sometimes from the first, an eruption of pimples or fever blisters appears around the mouth or lips, which are often very annoying.

TREATMENT.—When a cold begins with cough, sneezing, pain in the breast, and general feeling as from having taken cold, resort at once to the Specific No SEVEN, of which take two pellets dry, and repeat it every two hours.

If the cold commences with more severe symptoms, and some fever and considerable irritation of the lungs or bronchia, commence with Specific No. ONE and take two pellets every hour at first, and after a few hours continue them in alternation with No. SEVEN at intervals of two hours, and so continue the two remedies until the force of the disease is broken, when the No. SEVEN, will complete the cure.

Should the disease assume more the catarrhal form, affecting the eyes, nose and throat, the Specifics No. NINETEEN and No. SEVEN are the proper remedies, and should be administered as above.

In all cases of colds, drink freely of cold water, live somewhat abstemiously, avoid coffee, stimulants, over-feeding and exposure and fatigue.

## LARYNGITIS—INFLAMMATION OF THE LARYNX

We distinguish two forms of this disease, the one acute and running its course in a comparatively short time; the other chronic, which may continue for months or years. The acute form is characterized by hoarseness or a low, dull voice, or a difficult, whispering voice, wanting in modulation ; a sense of soreness or of tightness in the larynx and upper part of the chest ; difficult, tight or wheezing inspiration ; sensation of constriction in the throat, and inability to breathe freely accompanied with pain, whcih is increased by pressure on the protuberance of the throat, or along the larynx. There is usually a hoarse, muffled cough, sometimes convulsive and dry, or with expectoration of tough adhesive mucus, sensation as if there were a foreign body or lump in the throat. If the inflammation involves the pharynx, there will be difficulty and pain in swallowing. There is more or less fever, and increased redness on looking into the throat. In some cases the fever runs so high, and the hoarseness and difficulty of breathing are so great, as to approximate a case of true croup. But, as the treatment is similar, the fear of confounding the two diseases need occasion no embarassment.

TREATMENT.—In all serious, acute cases, the Specifics No. ONE and No. THIRTEEN should be dissolved in water, twelve pellets of each in six spoonfuls of water, in separate glasses, and of these give alternately every hour until the fever has abated, when the No. SEVEN may be substituted for the No. ONE, and these two last may be continued until the disease is arrested.

## CHRONIC LARYNGITIS—LARYNGEAL CONSUMPTION.

This chronic inflammation of the larynx, in some of its forms, is almost daily met with. It forms the so-called ministers' sore throat, and presents every grade of severity, from slight hoarseness and irritation, down through all shades of inflammation and ulceration, to the most inveterate forms of laryngeal consumption. The disease often commences with slight hoarseness and irritation of the throat, frequent hehming or raising of scanty mucus and slight cough. As the disease progresses, these symptoms increase, and there is also dryness, burning, itching or tickling and tightness, or in some cases a dull, smarting, or an acute pain in the larynx. The voice may be hoarse or whispering, or piping, and only formed with effort. In the earlier stages, the voice is uncertain and often breaks in singing or loud speaking. The cough, at first dry and short, becomes gradually loose, with raising of mucus or purulent expectoration. Gradually, as the disease progresses, ulceration takes place, generally marked by pain in the throat as from a sharp-pointed body, especially when speaking. Should the disease involve the pharynx, there is also difficulty in swallowing, and in the effort the food or drink may be returned through the nostrils. If the ulceration involves the rim of the glottis, the voice is lost and the patient only speaks in whispers. As ulceration progresses, the discharge becomes purulent, bloody and even offensive; portions of lymph, cartilage and even ossific matter are discharged; the cough and difficulty of deglutition increase, often in paroxysms; the general health gives way; hectic fever, night sweats, emaciation, swelling of the limbs, loss of appetite, vomiting with the cough, and diarrhœa, are unfavorable indications, and lead us to look for the worst. There is usually soreness of the larynx on pressure, and from the inhalation of cold air. Coughing, sneezing, speaking, laughing or swallowing frequently bring on a fit of severe suffering.

TREATMENT.—In the earlier stages, while there is simply hoarseness and some degree of dryness or irritation in the throat and cough, the Specific No. SEVEN will be sufficient to control it, and may be given two pellets at a time, and repeated every three or four hours, and so continued from day to day.

Should the hoarseness be more decided, with cough, dryness, heat and irritation of the throat, or if the disease is fairly developed, resort to the Specific No. THIRTEEN, of which give two pellets, dissolved in water, every three hours, and so continue for two or three days. After that, give the Nos. SEVEN and THIRTEEN in alternation, every three hours which may be given until the disease is cured.

Should there be decided fever, a dose or two of Specific No. ONE may be occasionally interposed with advantage.

## ACUTE BRONCHITIS OF CHILDREN—CATARRH OF THE BREAST—LUNG FEVER.

This disease consists of an acute inflammation of the lining membrane of the air passages. The inflammation may be limited to a portion of the bronchia, or involve the entire membrane, and it may be but slight and easily arrested, or it may be from the very first a very serious and dangerous malady. In young children, it is particularly dangerous, forming the so-called "lung fever," and the younger the child the more critical the attack. In adults, the disease is manifested by chilliness, succeeded by fever, hoarseness, difficult respiration, frequent severe and distressing cough, at first dry and later with expectoration of viscid, frothy mucus, which becomes copious and may be streaked with blood; oppression or sense of constriction of the chest; foul tongue, loss of appetite, debility, rapid pulse and increasing difficulty of breathing; pale lips, anxious countenance, a crepitation, whistling, rattling or droning in the chest becoming very sensible on applying the ear to its surface.

As the patient improves, the respiration becomes easier and more free, and the fever abates; expectoration becomes whiter, thicker, easier and less abundant. On the contrary, unfavorable symptoms are: increased difficulty of breathing; face becomes more and more livid, and is covered with perspiration; mucus accumulates more and more in the air-passages; the cough becomes feeble and fails to free the lungs of the accumulation; the mind wanders, and the patient is carried off.

In children, of an early age, it is quite frequent, and commences usually with symptoms of an ordinary cold; but soon the breathing becomes quick, oppressed and labored, and from the increased action of the diaphragm, the abdomen becomes prominent; the shoulders and nostrils are in continual motion from the effort of breathing; on applying the ear to the chest, and often at quite a distance from the patient, the *crepitation* and mucus-rattle of the chest is very audible; expectoration coughed into the mouth and then swallowed, temporarily relieves, and occasionally the mucus is thrown from the air-passages by the effort of vomiting; the cough is frequent, short and distressing; the face becomes pale, anxious, and somewhat livid. The disease has its paroxysms and seasons of remission, during which the child appears drowsy, and, unless relieved, the paroxysms recur with increasing severity until death takes place from suffocation. There is no appetite, but considerable thirst, and the symptoms are generally worse at night. Children at the breast find it difficult to nurse, from the oppression of the chest and impeded respiration.

TREATMENT.—The Specifics No. ONE and No. SEVEN are the proper remedies, and may be administered in fluid form as follows: If the symptoms are at all urgent, prepare the medicine for children of two years or under, by placing eight pellets of Specific No. ONE in as many teaspoonfuls of water, in one glass, and the same quantity of Specific

No. SEVEN in like quantity of water in another glass, then from these two give a spoonful every hour in alternation. Older children, or adults, may take twice as much at a dose as the above. In milder cases, a dose of two pellets every two hours may be sufficient, and these may be continued until the disease is arrested.

If in children, who are in far the most danger in this disease, the fever should have been allayed, but the cough and difficulty of breathing, attended with great weakness, remains, then omit the Specific No. ONE, and in place give the Specific No. SIX, the same dose, in alternation with No. SEVEN, and continue these so long as they are beneficial.

## PLEURISY.

This disease is of rather frequent occurrence, and is usually one of grave importance. It is an inflammation of the pleura or membrane, covering the lungs on one side, and being reflected upon the walls of the chest upon the other side, thus forms what is termed the pleural-sac. It is a very thin membraneous tissue, having a serous surface and quite liable to inflammation and consequent exudation of serum. The inflammation and pain may be located in any part of the chest, or even affect a considerable portion of it. A well marked pleurisy commences with a decided chill, lasting often some hours, followed by high fever, heat, red face, sharp, quick pulse, and *very severe stitching, stabbing* or *lancinating pains,* often confined to one spot in the side, or front of the chest. The pain is sharp, catching, lancinating, arresting or intercepting the breathing, and is greatly aggravated by coughing or even by movement; and the chest is *sensitive to pressure* at the *place where the pain is located.* The respiration is difficult and anxious, often intercepted by the stitch, but less oppressed than in pneumonia. The cough is short and dry, and greatly increases the stitch or pain in the side. The pulse is quick and hard; tongue inclined to dryness or parched; thirst decided; urine scanty and high-colored; and the patient generally lying on his back. If effusion of serum has occurred in one side of the chest, lying upon the opposite side is very difficult. The effusion is generally absorbed in the process of cure, but, when the absorbent powers of the system have become weakened, and the cure is imperfect, the secretion may be only partially taken up, and adhesion of the pleural surfaces may occur, thus practically uniting the surface of the lung to the walls of the chest, and occasioning more or less inconvenience in after life.

TREATMENT.—The Specifics No. ONE and No. SEVEN are the proper remedies, and should be given thus: Dissolve twelve pellets of No. ONE in as many spoonfuls of water, and of this give a spoonful (large if for an adult, and small if for a child) every half hour, and continue this medicine until the pulse is reduced and softened, the pain is diminished and the surface cooled, and for twenty-four hours, unless the disease has yielded before this period. Then prepare Specific No. SEVEN in like manner, and administer it in alternation with No. ONE, at intervals at first of one hour, and then at two hours, until the entire disease has succumbed.

In some rare cases, where the fever has been subdued, and some degree of pain in the chest or soreness yet lingers, the use of Specific No. FIFTEEN, either alone or in alternation with No. SEVEN, may remove it.

P. S. ☞ In pleurisy and inflammation of the lungs, or of other noble organ, if the attack is decided or well marked, it is advisable to give the patient at once a hot foot-bath in the manner recommended on page 43 of this work, so as to induce a determination of blood to the extremities, and excite general perspiration. After the patient has been put to bed, should the pain or breathing, and the oppression of the chest be severe, a hot fomentation, applied directly to the part, will be of great advantage. The best mode of making it is thus: Take common muslin, and cut out and run up a bag—say eight or ten by twelve inches—enough to entirely cover the suffering part. Fill this with meal and bran, in proportion of one part of meal to two of bran, so that when the filling shall be evenly distributed, the fomentation shall be about a half an inch or more in thickness. Pour say half an inch of hot water into a tin pan, and lay the bag in evenly spread out. It will at once become thoroughly hot and saturated, and may be applied directly to the chest as hot as can be borne, and covered with a flannel to prevent wetting the clothes. It rarely fails to afford prompt and decided relief, and may be repeated from time to time, if necessary, and is far better than blisters or mustard plasters.

## PLEURODYNIA—FALSE PLEURISY—STITCH IN THE SIDE.

This is a rheumatic affection of the intercostal muscles of the chest, and similar to pleurisy, in that it is characterized by a sharp stitch or stinging pain in the chest. It may be distinguished from pleurisy in *not* being preceded by a chill, and being without fever. The pain shifts from place to place. The surface of the chest or side is usually sore, and the pain may be excited by drawing the finger along between the ribs. A few doses of two pellets of Specific No. One or No. Fifteen will generally cure it, and they may be repeated every two hours.

## INFLAMMATION OF THE LUNGS—PNEUMONIA.

Inflammation of the substance of the lungs may occur alone, or in connection with pleurisy, which is indeed its most common form. It commences like pleurisy, with a chill, frequent rigors passing over the body for some hours, followed by fever, with great heat of the surface, which is hot and dry; pulse quick, but rarely so quick or bounding as in pleurisy; breathing is quickened, hot,oppressed, anxious, and sometimes interrupted by the pain; tongue dry, sometimes parched; urine high colored and scanty; cough short, distressing, and dry at first, gradually becomes more moist, raising a little adhesive viscid, or tenacious mucus, which is at first semi-transparent, but soon becomes greyish, mixed with blood, rust colored, or even like prune juice; the speech is interrupted, hesitating, with frequent pause and abdominal respiration. Sometimes the pain is not sharp, only dull, with a sense of oppression or tightness. The face is less red bnt more livid than in pleurisy; the vessels of the neck become swelled and turgid, and the frequent cough often causes severe headache. The patient lies upon his back, dislikes to talk and desires to be let alone; sometimes is very irritable or careless of his situation.

As the patient improves, the heat of the surface is reduced; the breathing is more free; the skin and tongue become and remain moist; the sputa becomes more free, less tenacious and lighter colored, and the cough less frequent and painful, and quiet sleep, with general perspiration and free discharge of urine, indicate a crisis and the breaking up of the disease. On the contrary, increased oppression of the chest, dryness of tongue and skin, frequency of the cough and scanty viscid, rust, expectoration, hiccough and delirium, indicate the progress of the disease. It is, however, generally curable in its earlier stages, under our management.

Treatment.—Should be commenced with Specific No. One, of which give two pellets, dissolved in water, every hour for the first twenty-four hours; also, give the patient a hot foot-bath, and if the tightness, oppression of the chest or pain is very severe, apply the hot fomentation to the chest, as directed under the treatment of pleurisy. After twenty-four hours, proceed to give the Specific No. SEVEN, prepared in the same manner as No. ONE, and give the two medicines in alternation, at intervals of one hour. Continue this until the disease is removed, gradually increasing the intervals between the doses to two or even three hours, as the improvement progresses.

After convalescence, should there remain some tendency to cough, debility and sweating at night, two pellets of No. TEN at night, and of No. THIRTY-FIVE each morning, rarely fail to complete the cure.

## CONGESTION OF THE CHEST.

This condition, determination of blood to the chest, may be supposed to exist where there is a sensation of fulness, heaviness, weight or oppression in the chest. There may be also throbbings, or palpitations of the heart, attended with anxiety, short, sighing, or difficult breathing, and sometimes a short cough. It is most common in young plethoric subjects, or those of consumptive habit. It is sometimes occasioned by over exertion, exposure to heat and cold, use of stimulants, coffee, spices, vinous or alcoholic beverages, or may be caused by suppression of eruptions or accustomed discharges.

TREATMENT.—In general a few doses of Specific No. ONE, two pellets, taken at intervals of one or two hours, will promptly relieve it. Should there be frequent recurrence of the attack, or the condition threatens to become chronic, administer the Specific No. THIRTY-FIVE each night on retiring, and the No. ONE each morning. If it has been caused by suppression, or too scanty flow of the menses, give the Specific No. ELEVEN, and repeat every two hours until relieved. If connected with constipation, hemorrhoid or indigestion, administer the Specific No. TEN in like manner.

## ASTHMA.

This affection of the lungs and air passages is characterized by difficulty of breathing, coming on in paroxysms, attended with a suffocative, or constrictive sensation, cough and expectoration. The paroxysms may come on suddenly, without warning, and more frequently at night, but often they are preceded by a feeling of irritation in the air passages, or a sense of fulness or oppression at the pit of the stomach. During the attack the respiration is labored, wheezing or sighing long drawn, accompanied with anxiety, and the shoulders, larynx and chest are moved with the violence of the effort. The patient usually sits or stands, can rarely recline, and his arms elevated so as to expand to the chest; often requires the doors or windows to be opened to give him air. There is a sense of constriction or tightness in the chest, or as if he was breathing through a sponge; frequent cough, at first short, dry, then, by degrees, becoming more moist; or with frequent profuse expectoration of mucus, even from the first; the face is pale, sometimes livid; eyes anxious and protruded; often cold sweat on the forehead, face and chest; often palpitation of the heart or arteries, and the pulse is irregular, quick or intermittent. These paroxysms last from a few hours to as many days, and recur again in a few days or weeks, leaving the patient comparatively free in the interval. It is common to divide the disease into two varieties,—the dry and moist asthma. In the first the attacks are more sudden, and cough short, dry, with little expectoration, even towards its close; while in the latter, the attack is more gradual and the cough more severe, and the expectoration becomes copious, as relief is afforded.

The disease may arise from a variety of morbid conditions, such as chronic induration, or extreme irritability of the mucus membrane of the air passages; disease of the heart, or large vessels, or similar organic changes. The paroxysms are frequently excited by exposure, a chill, the use of stimulants, or indigestion.

TREATMENT.—Our success in curing this disease depends upon our ability to remove the morbid condition from whence it arises. In some cases, the medicines directed will perfectly meet the indication, and so a permanent cure will be effected. In others it may be in its nature incurable, and in these cases we are only able to palliate the disease, or fundamental condition, and to relieve the attacks when they recur.

During the interval, and to prevent a recurrence of the attack, take two pellets of the Specific No. TWENTY-ONE at night, and two of No. SEVEN each morning, unless some particular demand be made for some other medicine, for some other symptom or indication. During the paroxysm, dissolve twelve pills of Specific No. TWENTY-ONE in six spoonfuls of water, and of these give one every hour, and so continue until the paroxysm has abated, gradually prolonging the intervals as the amendment progresses.

If there is palpitation, or violent beating of the heart, you may give in alternation with No. TWENTY-ONE, the Specific No. THIRTY-TWO. Sometimes very violent paroxysms have been relieved by Specific No. SIX, given in like manner. Children require only half the above doses.

## PULMONARY HEMORRHAGE, HÆMOPTYSIS. BLEEDING FROM THE LUNGS.

This is always a very grave affection, sometimes very dangerous indeed. Not more so from what it is in itself than from the condition of the pulmonary tissue which it indicates. The bleeding may arise from one of several conditions: Thus, it may arise as a mere exudation from the mucus surface of the lungs, bronchia or throat; or from congestion or engorgement and overfilling of the vessels and substance of the lungs; or it may arise from a rupture of one or more important, or of numerous minute blood-vessels in the substance of the lungs. Thus, in any case, it points to a morbid and more or less critical condition of the pulmonary organs. The first and second forms mentioned are generally curable, and the cure of the last depends upon our ability to control or cure the general disease. All blood thrown from the mouth is not necessarily from the lungs. Sometimes it comes from the stomach, but in this case it is vomited up—comes up with retching and nausea, in quantities, and is of dark color, while if it comes from the lungs, it comes with coughing or hehming, and is lighter colored, or bright red, or frothy,—comes with a hot or boiling sensation, or sense of effervescence in the chest, the patient often knowing just where it comes from, and it is generally attended with great sinking and prostration of strength.

Bleeding from the lungs sometimes comes on as the vicarious effect of a suppression of the menses, or other discharge, and is cured with the restoration of the suppressed function. It occasionally occurs in stout, full-blooded, plethoric individuals, and is of less consequence than when it occurs in spare, meagre, consumptive individuals.

TREATMENT.—When a hemorrhage occurs, it is all important that the patient and all the attendants should be calm and discreet, not rash or hasty. Noise, haste and fright are the most dangerous auxiliaries of the accident, while composure and presence of mind are half the battle.

The patient should be placed as quietly as possible in a half-sitting or reclining position, and be perfectly at rest, without speaking or being spoken to, having his wants anticipated if possible. Supply the patient with cloths or a vessel, so he may discharge the blood from the mouth, without effort of the body. If a good Homeopathic physician is at hand, let him be sent for.

If you have HUMPHREYS' WITCH HAZEL, get it at

once, and put a large spoonful into a common drinking glass, half full of water, and of this give a dessert spoonful every five, ten or fifteen minutes, according to the effect, being careful to prolong the intervals to half an hour, one or two hours, in proportion as the bleeding is arrested. It will act very promptly if the blood is a little dark, not bright red. If you have not the WITCH HAZEL, use a tablespoonful of common salt, with the same quantity of water, and give in the same manner.

If the *blood is more red and frothy*, and especially with young, plethoric individuals, put twenty pellets of the Specific No. ONE in the quantity of water mentioned above, and give a dessert spoonful at the intervals above mentioned, *in alternation* with the *W. Hazel.* These remedies will very generally arrest the hemorrhage, yet the patient should, for some days, be exceedingly careful to avoid effort, coughing, exertion, or exposure, to prevent a recurrence of the attack. To prevent fever, or an inflammatory condition of the lungs, after hemorrhage, or the development of consumption, give the Specifics No. ONE and No. SEVEN, two pellets every three hours, in alternation, gradually prolonging the intervals, until they are taken only four times in the day, before each meal and on going to rest at night, which may be continued until the health is restored.

When, after a hemorrhage from the lungs, a *soreness* of the *chest* or *any part* of it remains, wet a napkin or smaller thin cloth, large enough to cover the chest or affected place, in WITCH HAZEL, and lay this on over the part, covering it again well with a dry flannel, which may be continued over night, or even be worn with advantage through the day.

## PULMONARY CONSUMPTION—PHTHISIS PULMONALIS.

Consumption is one of the most frequent and fatal diseases to which the human family are subject. It prevails in all countries and in all climates, and among all classes, the poor and the rich, the well and ill-cared for. It is doubtless less in some countries and climates than others, but none has yet been found which is exempt from it. So of classes and conditions of society. None have been found among whom this disease is a stranger. The most nearly exempt are those families who for years have exclusively used appropriate and properly prepared (potentised) Homeopathic medicines. For I think it demonstrable, that proper Homeopathic medication tends to destroy and eliminate from the system the tuberculous diathesis, which is the foundation of this disease. True, consumption may come from numerous morbid conditions, which, by exhausting or debilitating the system, produce that condition of innervation, or vital prostration, during which only tubercles are deposited; so that these diseases or conditions have been only the stepping stone to the tuberculous deposit and consumption itself.

This disease may approach in several different ways, some of which we will indicate. It is most common among subjects from seventeen to twenty-five years of age. It is perceptibly lessened at thirty-five, and over fifty quite unusual. In the more insidious form, the patient may be noticed to have a little less vigor and energy than usual; to have less of flesh or embonpoint; lips and cheeks a little paler than usual; complains of being out of breath on exercise, or has even a slight tightness on breathing; has a little dry cough or a hack, as it is called, and may raise a little frothy mucus. These symptoms may go on for months, without attracting particular attention, or pass off altogether, and then recur again. If not arrested, the cough gradually grows more frequent, dry, irritating, troubling the patient, especially at night; the loss of flesh becomes more manifest, while the appetite may be yet fair, or only capricious; gradually there is some chilliness in the morning hours, and some heat towards evening; the cheeks are more pale, and the fingers more attenuated, and the ends of the nails somewhat hooked; by degrees the cough becomes more frequent, expectoration more abundant, white, frothy and streaked with yellow, and may be saltish or sweetish to the taste; chills now become more decided, recurring every day, usually in the morning, with heat, and circumscribed redness of cheeks every afternoon; the bowels, until now confined, become loose, with frequent stools; sweat comes on at night, at first around the neck and chest, greasy or sticky, and gradually over the entire person; the cough, expectoration and emaciation progress more and more; the feet and legs swell; the mind wanders, and death gradually closes the scene. The pulse is a pretty good indication, and becomes frequent, quite early in the disease, and gradually increases from 70 to 80, and then to 120 beats to the minute.

In some cases consumption comes on as the sequel to other diseases. These being imperfectly cured, leave the system exhausted, and tubercles are deposited, which, beginning to soften, produce irritation, cough, pain in the chest or side, quick pulse, hectic fever, emaciation, night sweats, diarrhœa, expectoration of pus, or yellow, heavy, thick, adhesive mucus, and all the usual symptoms attending the advanced stage of this disease. Ladies, after confinement, not unfrequently run into consumption after this fashion. Yet, on looking back over the history of the case, it will be found that there had existed previously, some cough, pain in the side, or oppression of the chest, emaciation or debility, which was in fact the premonitory stage of the disease, and which was suspended for a time, and only warmed into vigor by the debility occasioned by the new attack of disease.

In some subjects, especially those in early life and of peculiar temperaments, the disease runs so rapid a course, as to have secured the name of "galloping consumption." This is especially so with persons of scrofulous habit, viz: Thin, light skin, fair hair, long teeth, waxen complexion, tall stature, or with thin chest and pointed shoulders, and enlarged glands beneath the cheek or along the sides of the neck. Not unfrequently such individuals, with few or no premonitions, beyond a slight cough and some degree of debility and weakness, a slight or severe hemorrhage from the lungs occurs, by which the strength of the patient is cut down at once, and in comparatively few days, cough, expectoration and hectic fever set in, and the patient runs along the course of the consumption with rapid strides.

Advanced cases of consumption are easily recognized; the earlier stages, the incipient beginnings are readily overlooked, and, but too frequently, grave mischief has been done before the patient or friends have been aware of danger. But whenever a person has some slight or severe cough, which does not pass off readily, some shortness or tightness of breath, or pain in the chest or side, and above all, if she is feeble, easily fatigued and *emaciated*, or losing flesh, it is better to give ourselves the advantage of the doubt, and at once apply the remedies and means for a cure, rather than wait the farther development of the disease.

THE CURABILITY of consumption is a mooted question, and one upon which popular impression and medical testimony are at variance. But I hold the moderate view of the cure to be this: That all cases of incipient or undeveloped consumption are easily curable, by proper remedies and appropriate surroundings. That cases in the second stage have a fair chance of recovery, while in the more advanced cases the recoveries are only rare.

TREATMENT.—As the earliest and perhaps most striking symptom is the cough, all that has been said in the chapter, upon that subject, is applicable here. In the earlier stages of the disease, the Specific No. SEVEN is the appropriate remedy. But should there be fever, or some heat of surface on the palms of the hands, or some pain or soreness in the chest or sides, the Specific No. ONE may be given in alternation with it, at intervals of two or three hours, two pellets at a time. Should the case have made considerable progress, with hard, racking cough, considerable expectoration and some emaciation, and especially in scrofulous subjects, the Specifics No. THIRTY-FIVE and No. SEVEN should be given in alternation, at intervals of three or four hours.

If the patient is confined to the house or room, the medicine had best be given in solution, in the proportion of two pellets in a spoonful of water, of which a spoonful should be given at a time. But if the patient is yet around, the pellets may be taken dry.

IN THE TREATMENT of this disease, too much stress cannot be laid upon the diet, habits and surroundings of the patient, as the disease is essentially one of debility, effecting not only his nutrition, but also the revivification of the blood, by the atmospheric air, it is all important, in the process of cure, that these two indications be fully met. Hence, the patient should have a diet the most nourishing and easily digested possible, such as cream, milk if it agrees; good bread, not too new; good fresh butter; puddings of Indian, wheat, rye, oatmeal or rice; all succulent and ripe fruits in their season, unless they produce diarrhœa. Use meat and meat soups, without spices, in moderation; beef, mutton, poultry, venison, game, small birds. For beverage, cold water, cocoa, black tea, and some good, light, native or pure foreign wine, once or twice per day. In cases where good wine cannot be had, good whisky is to be recommended, in portions from a dessert spoonful to a wineglass, oft-repeated experience that the use of stimulants in the treatment of consumption is indispensable, and I have succeeded in curing many patients by this procedure, who, I am satisfied, could otherwise never have been saved. The quantity commenced with should be small, and may be increased as the appetite, strength, and tone of the system improves.

The apartment of the patient should be high, dry, large and airy, and the temperature in winter or rough weather kept as uniform as possible, or at least, free from extremes, and he should have all the out-door air possible. If the patient is sufficiently vigorous, walking and horseback exercise are best, but in general, daily or constant rides in carriage are the preferable modes, and of these in good weather, the patient can scarcely have too much up to the point of fatigue. Changes of location whether South or North, inland or seaward, are always beneficial, provided we do not leave home comforts for the vexations and exposures almost necessarily incident to travel.

# DISEASES OF THE CIRCULATORY SYSTEM.

## ANGINA PECTORIS.—STENOCARDIA.

This disease most commonly attacks persons who have passed the meridian of life. It is also most common among literary men, or those subject to long continued mental effort, anxiety or disquietude. It is not always manifested in the same manner or with the same symptoms, but in general, it is known by a sudden attack of extreme agitation in the chest, generally referred by the patient to his heart; coming on suddenly and without premonition; attended by a feeling of constriction or suffocation, so that the patient, if walking, is at once compelled to stop, or if standing, to sink down; the first attack most commonly comes on during walking, or some severe effort; but afterwards the most trivial exercise, excitement, or mental effort, or even indigestible food, will produce them; and they finally come on suddenly without any assignable cause, and even while in bed and asleep. There is in most instances severe and sometimes excruciating pains, at first comfined to the chest, but afterwards extending to the shoulders, and sometimes along both the upper extremities. These paroxysms frequently terminate in a few minutes, leaving the patient comparatively free, and return again at uncertain intervals; while in other cases, they last some hours, or indeed, rarely leave the patient free from severe pain. In severe cases, the suffering is extreme, the face becomes pale and haggard, with an expression of extreme anguish, the eyes sunken, nose pointed, surface cold, and even cold clammy sweats, respiration difficult and rapid, palpitation or intermitting pulsation of the heart, anxiety or feeling of approaching

10

death; the pulse may be quick, strong and irregular, with hot skin and flushed face, but is most frequently slow, feeble, oppressed and remittent. Sometimes the attack passes off, leaving no trace, but commonly soreness about the chest remains for quite a period, and the digestion is more or less impaired. The duration and result of the disease are uncertain, and the pathological conditions upon which it is founded, vary in different cases.

TREATMENT.—For stout, plethoric, full-fed persons, the Specific No. ONE is most efficient, and should be resorted to at once, and may be given, dissolved in a spoonful of water, in doses of two pellets, repeated every half hour, or even every ten minutes, if the suffering is severe. Should the patient not be relieved after an hour, give the Specific No. THIRTY-TWO in the same manner, and repeat at intervals of half an hour until relief is afforded. For any remaining suffering, give the two Specifics No. ONE and No. THIRTY-TWO, in alternation, at intervals of one, two or three hours, according to the urgency of the case.

To prevent a repetition of the attack, give the Specific No. THIRTY-TWO, two pellets at a dose, morning and night, either dry on the tongue or dissolved in water, as may be most convenient.

## CARDITIS—ENDOCARDITIS—PERICARDITIS.

*Inflammation of the substance of the heart, inflammation of the lining membrane of the heart, and inflammation of the investing membrane of the heart—*

It is preferable to treat these diseases in connection in a work designed for domestic practice. Systematic writers detail at length the symptoms and diognostic signs by which they may be distinguished, but the non-professional reader would be unable to make these distinctions, and would find it impossible to base a treatment upon them. He can at best only expect to ascertain that some portion of the heart is the subject of inflammatory action, and to apply general remedies adapted for its cure in the absence of competent medical aid. In some cases the symptoms are, at least for a time, masked and insidious, and in others more decided and marked; but in general we may conclude that some form of inflammatory disease of the heart exists, from the presence of the following symptoms:—

Sharp, burning, prickling or darting pains in the region of the heart, attended with fever. The pains shoot to the left shoulder and shoulder blade, and frequently extend along the arm; they are aggravated by deep inspiration, and are increased by pressure on the spaces between the ribs in the region of the heart. The patient cannot lie on the left side, but finds the position easiest on the back; breathing is rapid, irregular and laborious, especially on movement; a feeling of contraction, restlessness, anxiety and frequent faintness. The pulse is accelerated, at times hard, full and vibratory; then again, feeble, irregular or intermittent, while if the ear is applied to the region of the heart, its action will be found to be tremulous and violent, sometimes again it is found to be muffled, veiled and indistinct, indicating an effusion of lymph within the pericardium or investing membrane of the heart. Sometimes the sounds seem double, prolonged, rough, or even blowing or grating, from defective action of the valves. In all cases, the impulse of the heart against the walls of the chest will be found more violent than in health. If extensive effusion has taken place around the heart, the extremities will generally become œdematous or enlarged.

TREATMENT.—So far as it can be conducted without competent professional aid, consists in the Specifics No. ONE and No. THIRTY-TWO. They should be given alternately, dissolved in water, ten pellets at a time, at intervals of from one to three hours. according to the urgency of the symptoms. After the more immediate attack has passed, the Specific No. THIRTY-TWO should be continued for some time, repeated morning and night, to remove and correct any remaining morbid action.

In case of effusion within the pericardium, indicated by œdema of the extremities or predominent suffocation sensation, the Specific No. TWENTY-FIVE may be given with advantage, repeated every two hours.

## PALPITATION OF THE HEART.

This affection may arise from a variety of causes. Young people, when rapidly growing, are liable to it, likewise the aged, as it may arise from an excess or deficient supply of blood. Nervous persons, from a peculiar habit of body, are disposed to it. Ardent spirits and the use of strong coffee or green tea produce it in some cases, especially in those of sedentary habits. Many persons, when suffering from indigestion, have palpitation or irregular action of the heart. Pregnant females, and those at the change of life, are very commonly affected with it. In all these cases it may be merely functional and disappear with the occasioning cause. There are also other cases in which it depends upon organic changes in the structure of the heart itself, its valvular apparatus, or the large vessels immediately connected with it, and where the use of medicine can have but a subordinate effect in relieving it.

TREATMENT.—In general, a dose of two pellets of Specific No. ONE, repeated every hour, if need be, speedily removes it. Should the No. ONE fail, the Specific No. THIRTY-TWO may be resorted to in like manner, and will rarely fail to afford relief. Should the palpitation arise from indigestion, that complaint being relieved by Specific No. TEN, the palpitation or irregular action of the heart will cease, or may be speedily controlled by the No. THIRTY-TWO. When it arises in connection with scanty, delayed or interrupted menses, the Specific No. ELEVEN, two pills, four times per day, will relieve.

## CHRONIC DISEASE OF THE HEART.

There are various structural alterations of the heart or some portions of it, or of its complicated apparatus, such as enlargements in various directions, thickening or thinning of its walls, defects of its valvular structure, aneurism or dilatation of its larger vessels, etc., all of which give rise to various symptoms and inconveniencies, and are more or less critical, according to the nature of the case. With some of these cardiac changes, the patients live on for years and with ease, and scarcely suffer more than inconvenience, while others have a constant sense of oppression, shortness of breath at exercise, mounting stairs or mental emotion, constant palpitation or labored action of the heart, difficulty in lying with the head low, and, not unfrequently, pain in the region of the heart or chest, or along the left arm.

It would be impracticable here to describe these various cases and the treatment appropriate to each, and such had best be submitted to competent medical examination. But in the absence of a good Homeopathic physician, the patient may take with great relief and often with permanent advantage, the Specific No. THIRTY-TWO, two pellets at a time, and may repeat them two, three or more times per day, according to the urgency of the case. Often, under such treatment, very grave diseases of the heart are wonderfully modified and controlled, and the life of the patient prolonged and rendered useful and comfortable.

## VARICOSE VEINS.

Not unfrequently, the veins, especially of the lower extremities, becomes enlarged, knotted, dark-blue, or purple, sometimes the size of the finger or larger, and are termed *varicose veins.* They are very apt to occur in women during pregnancy, and in men of hemorrhoidal or venous habit of body, and especially in those whose occupation requires constant standing on the feet. The varicose veins are generally painless, but sometimes are attended with burning, shooting or stinging pains, and at times terminate in indolent, obstinate ulcers, or sometimes occasion general œdema of the limbs.

TREATMENT.—If the varices are not specially troublesome, bathing them at night with WITCH HAZEL will allay any pain or irritation, and the Specific No. THIRTY-TWO, two pellets, may be taken morning and night.

For their radical cure and removal, an *elastic stocking* should be worn from the arch of the foot well up over the enlarged veins, and each morning and night the part should be bathed in WITCH HAZEL, or yet better, a cloth wet with the same and laid on over the enlarged veins, and the stocking turned over that, and so worn, while the medicine above directed may be taken internally. This course will promptly relieve and ultimately restore even the most formidable cases.

# DISEASES OF THE ALIMENTARY TRACK.

## SORE THROAT—QUINSY.

This disease is quite common, some persons being subject to it from the slightest provocation or exposure. It usually commences with a sensation of tightness or constriction, or a sensation of a lump or plug in the throat, and some soreness manifested, particularly in the act of swallowing; as the disease progresses, the deglutition becomes more painful and difficult, the root of the tongue, the tonsils, the curtains of the palate, and adjoining soft parts, become swelled, red and painful. There is considerable thirst, fever, pulse quick and strong; the tongue becomes coated and breath offensive, heat of the surface, red cheeks, eyes sometimes inflamed, headache, and even delirium. In some cases the throat is so swelled that deglutition becomes almost impossible, the fluid returning through the nose, and the throat, where it can be seen, is the seat of more or less extensive ulceration. In some cases these ulcers are superficial, and confined to slight suppuration of the tonsils; in others they involve the soft parts, and the discharge, when it occurs, is quite extensive. When taken in time and properly treated, the disease disappears by resolution, otherwise it yields only when the abscess breaks. It more commonly affects only one side or one tonsil, sometimes passing over to the other, and is more serious when both are involved. It is not generally dangerous, but in some cases, and in particular epidemics, is liable to assume a putrid character with typhoid symptoms, and may then become a more dangerous malady.

Treatment.—At the commencement, when there is considerable heat, fever and pain on swallowing, the Specific No.

One, two pellets, should be given every hour, in a spoonful of water, for two or three times, and then the Specific No. Thirty-four should be prepared in the same manner, eight or ten pellets in six spoonfuls of water, and one spoonful be given every hour from the two medicines, in alternation, and so continued until the disease yields; only as the amendment progresses, the intervals between the doses may be prolonged to two hours, and finally to three or more. When there is simple soreness of the throat and pain on swallowing, without fever, the No. Thirty-four may be used from the first, and exclusively. In some cases, where the disease may have gone on to suppuration, and the discharge has taken place, and the pain and difficulty of deglutition diminished, only the ulcerative process is slow to heal, the use of Specific Nos. Twenty-two and Twenty-three may be given in alternation, in doses of two pellets, four times per day, until entire restoration.

## PUTRID OR MALIGNANT SORE THROAT.

This disease generally appears as an epidemic, often as a part of that scourge, the malignant scarlet fever. It is not often seen isolated, yet some cases of quinsy may assume some of its features.

It usually commences with shivering, followed by heat, and from the first there is decided languor and prostration; some oppression in breathing; nausea, and after, repeated vomiting and sometimes purging; eyes inflamed and watery; cheeks deep red color; tonsils become inflamed, throat bright red color and much swelled; thin, acrid discharge from the tonsils and throat, which excoriates the nose and lips; pulse weak, small and irregular, and scarcely perceptible; tongue white and moist, and swallowing very difficult. This condition soon changes, and ulcerations, varying in size and situation, appear upon the tonsils and surrounding soft parts, which, on inspection, are seen to be swelled and livid. These ulcerations may extend over the curtains of the palate and forward into the posterior portion of the mouth, or back down into the windpipe, and assume a sloughing or decomposed appearance as they increase in magnitude. The prostration of strength becomes more decided; the lips and teeth are covered with sordes or blackish incrustations; the breath becomes very offensive; there is more or less delirium; the countenance becomes sunken and there is some purging. Sometimes the entire neck becomes swelled and livid, and in some very severe cases livid spots or petecchiæ make their appearance on the surface of the body. Extreme prostration, bleedings from the nose and mouth, weak, fluttering, intermittent pulse, and appearance of livid spots, *petecchiæ,* mark the extreme violence and dangerous character of the disease.

When about the third or fourth day a gentle perspiration breaks out, and the sloughs are thrown off so as to leave a clean, healthy surface upon the ulcers in the throat, and the countenance brightens up, and the respiration and pulse become more natural, a favorable termination may be anticipated.

TREATMENT.—The Specifics No. ONE and No. THIRTY-FOUR should be given from the commencement and continued through the entire course of the disease. They may be given in alternation, a spoonful every hour, and during the height of the disease, every half hour.

Dissolve twelve pellets of each Specific in six spoonfuls of water, in separate glasses, and give to children a teaspoonful, and to adults a tablespoonful of the fluid in alternation, at the intervals above mentioned, and so continue, only omitting when the patient is quietly sleeping, and prolonging the intervals between the doses as the patient improves.

*Diet* and *Regimen.*—Rarely can patients suffering from this disease take much food of any description, and only that which has been divested of its rough or harsh particles can be allowed, such as rice-water, soft-boiled rice, toast-water, arrow root, farina, gum-water, corn-starch or thin flour gruel. When the mouth and lips become dry, or the sloughs dry and hard, the mouth and lips should be frequently and carefully moistened with warm milk and water. Care should be taken, when the patient begins to recover, that the stomach is not overloaded, lest painful after diseases may be provoked. Hence, begin moderately with rice, toast, black tea, cocoa, baked or stewed apples, milk-toast, and light soups, and only very gradually return to a more substantial diet.

## DIPHTHERIA.

This disease has of late years made terrible ravages in certain portions of the United States, and has come to be regarded as a much dreaded visitation. It is not a new disease, but has latterly attracted more attention, and probably assumed a more malignant and fatal form than in previous years. It is not considered as contagious, though the same influences that excite its attack in one member of a family are likely to exist in others, and so to invite its approach, and it is quite probable that the exciting causes of its attack are more potent in its immediate presence than at a distance. It commonly prevails in certain neighborhoods or sections of country, and to this extent may be said to be epidemic. It is one of those diseases which should rarely be entrusted to the care of even intelligent laymen, in an emergency, or in the absence of a competent Homeopathic physician; but in all severe cases, so soon as the nature of the disease is known, it should be handed over to the most skillful medical attendance, and his directions followed with fidelity. Sometimes Diphtheria is a light and easily-managed disease, while at others it is terribly fatal and runs its desolating course, paying but little attention to the best medical means devised for its arrest. Hence, every head of a family should be able to recognize its earlier symptoms and in an emergency to apply the most approved medicines for its cure.

Diphtheria generally prevails among children and young people, full adults being only occasionally attacked. Its earlier symptoms are like those of some other diseases, especially simulating mumps or scarlet fever. The child is at first languid and uneasy, with a pulse quickened but not extremely full, and is restless, without much appetite. These symptoms may continue for some days without any appearance of inflammation of the throat or fauces. In other cases the glands in front of and below the ear may enlarge, simulating mumps, or there may be stiffness of the muscles of the neck, or pains in the ears or in the limbs. As the disease advances, the want of appetite continues; sometimes there is vomiting; the pulse becomes quicker, but weaker. Upon examination the throat appears reddened and congested, and sometimes there is difficulty in deglutition, but this is by no means universal, as cases have been known where the disease was far advanced before this symptom was manifested. Should the evacuations be examined at this period, the stools will be frequently found covered with mucus, and the urine loaded with albuminous matter, severe periodical pains in the limbs are also present. An examination of the throat, which is in many instances a very difficult matter, owing to the patient's inability to sufficiently open the mouth, will exhibit patches of membranous exudation quite small, often at first not larger than a split pea, *whitish*, or of a *yellowish* or *tawny hue*, deposited mostly in the irregularities of tonsils, or in the arch of the palate or in both, and the tonsils are at times enormously swollen. Salivation, which may have commenced earlier in the progress of the disease, continues, the pulse is quick and the prostration of the system decided. If under the influence of the proper remedies, the disease is arrested and convalescence begins, it will be manifested by a sense of ease and quiet, refreshing slumber and free perspiration, diminution of the swelled glands, arrest of the membranous formation, and the gradual disappearance of that already existing, slower pulse and returning appetite.

In some cases, as the disease progresses, there may be no farther increase of the exudation in the throat, but a watery fluid is discharged from the nose, the eye becomes brighter, and countenance anxious; the breathing is labored and rattling, and worse when the patient attempts to sleep; the voice is impaired; the exudation has increased and even reached the roof of the mouth, with increasing prostration. Such cases are very severe, yet some from even this stage have recovered.

As the disease progresses, the difficult, stridulous breathing increases, and a hollow, croupy, metallic, whistling cough shows that the larynx is invaded. The discharge from the nose continues, and fluids taken into the mouth return by the nose. The cheeks have a pale, ashen hue, and there are some mottled or slightly congested spots. Periodical and severe pains occur in the limbs, hemorrhage from the nose and mouth may be very troublesome, and new and large patches of the exudation may be found upon the fauces. The difficulty of respiration increases, the patient grasps at the neck or clothing in the vain attempt to get air; the blueness of the face and surface increases, and death comes to close the scene. Or in some cases the swelling of the glands subside, the false membrane disappears from sight, and the patient sinks from the effects of the constitutional poison, and ultimately dies with scarcely a sigh or a groan.

There are several diseases which simulate and are liable to be mistaken for diphtheria, or indeed may appear in connection with it; or diphtheritic symptoms may be manifested in other diseases to which we call attention. First, and perhaps most important among these is scarlet fever. Sometimes diphtheria is accompanied with a rash, and as it may appear during or at the close of an epidemic of scarlet fever, and so be the more liable to be confounded with that disease. But the two diseases may in general be recognized by observing that the attack of scarlet fever is more sudden and that of diphtheria is more insidious; that the early swelling of the glands of the neck in diphtheria is out of all proportion to the soreness of the throat; and also to the intense pain in the head, high fever and very frequent pulse, which characterize the worst forms of diphtheria. After some hours, the decisive symptoms of the *false membrane in the throat, soft palate and uvula* will leave no doubt of the character of the enemy we have to deal with. In membranous croup we have the same false membrane as in diphtheria, but in croup it commences in the larynx and trachea, and only rarely extends up into the throat and fauces, while from the first the croupy cough, difficult breathing, and absence of swelling of the glands mark the disease as different from true diphtheria.

The premonitory symptoms of mumps—chilliness, fever, languor and want of appetite—are similar to those of diphtheria, and the swelling of the parotid and neighboring glands of the neck are much the same. The characteristic distinction lies in the presence of the false membrane before mentioned in the throat, and the hollow, barking, croupy cough, and difficult stridulous breathing, especially during sleep, which mark true diphtheria.

Treatment.—During the invasive stage, before the disease has been fully pronounced, it will of course be treated according to whatever symptoms should be most manifest, among which the remedies for *fever* and for *croup* will be prominent. But if diphtheria is prevalent, or there is reason to suspect it in the case presented, the Specific for this disease, No. THIRTY-FOUR, should be given, two pellets at a time, and repeated every two hours, either alone or in alternation with Specific No. ONE, especially if there should be any chilliness, fever, or unusual heat of the system.

During the prevalence of the disease, or when it has invaded a family, it is wise to administer two pellets of Specific No. THIRTY-FOUR each morning and night as a preventive, to the children who may be liable to an attack. The outbreak of the disease may thus be prevented altogether, or at least greatly modified and lessened in its violence.

When the disease has manifested itself with some degree of fever, swelling of the neck or glands, sore throat, whether it may be simple, or complicated with scarlatina, commence at once with the Specifics No. ONE and No. THIRTY-FOUR, and of these, two pellets should be administered in water every hour, in alternation. This course should be continued without variation or intermission except when the patient is in quiet sleep, when the interval may be prolonged until quiet waking affords opportunity for repeating the dose. The better mode is to dissolve twelve pellets of each Specific in six dessert spoonfuls of water, each in separate glasses, and of these administer in alternation as before directed. As the disease yields, the fever, heat, agitation, pain and swelling of the glands diminish, and a mild, profuse sweat breaks out over the system with quiet sleep, the case augurs a favorable termination, and the medicine may be given at rather longer intervals as the disease improves, and when the fever and heat has measurably disappeared, the Specific No. THIRTY-FOUR should only be given, administered as before in fluid, every hour.

The diet during the treatment of this disease is important and should consist mainly of beef-tea, or soup of venison, mutton or chicken, and of this the patient may be encouraged to take, from time to time, such quantities as the system requires or the little appetite permits. These animal soups are in this case preferable to rice, farina, or meal gruel, as they contribute less to the formation of the peculiar diphtheritic deposit, and sustain the system better.

## SCURVY OF THE MOUTH—CANKER SORE MOUTH.

This affection manifests itself in various forms, sometimes being quite severe and obstinate, and at others, more inconvenient and painful than dangerous. In some cases the gums become hot, red and very sensitive; they swell, become spongy, and shrink from the teeth, leaving them loose, and the gums readily bleeding at the slightest injury; the breath becomes offensive, and sometimes there is discharge of tough, sanious phlegm and saliva; mastication may become difficult from the loose, sensitive teeth, and deglutition painful from the soreness of the throat; the glands of the throat sometimes swell and become painful, and there is often great prostration and a torpid, feverish condition of the system.

In other cases the disease is principally manifested by apthous ulcers appearing upon the gums, the tongue, or the inside of the lips and cheeks, attended with a painful, burning, smarting sensation, and at times free flow of saliva, and a feverish, prostrated condition of the system. This form is very common with nursing mothers, and is often very painful and lingering, apparently arising from an exhausted or debilitated condition of the system and defective nutrition.

TREATMENT.—In general, the Specific No. TWENTY-NINE will be sufficient for all forms of sore mouth or apthous ulcerations in the mouth. It may conveniently be given, two pellets at a dose, dissolved in a spoonful of water, and administered four times per day, before meals and on retiring at night.

Where there is a prostrated or debilitated condition of the system, the Specific No. Twenty-four may be given to advantage, in alternation with No. Twenty-nine, at the intervals before directed. Sometimes a weak solution of borax and water may be used to advantage for rinsing the mouth. Sometimes the mouth may be rinsed with a weak solution of brandy and water, with benefit in bad cases with debilitated subjects. Some care should be exercised in regard to diet. When the disease exists in a bad form, with extensive inflammation of the mouth or gums, stimulants and animal food, even in soups, should be avoided, and the diet confined to farinaceous or vegetable forms of food. In cases of nursing sore mouth, a glass of ale morning and night may be used with advantage in connection with the Specifics mentioned.

## OFFENSIVE BREATH.

This unpleasant affection may be dependent upon other causes than decayed teeth or impurities in the mouth. Not unfrequently it arises from imperfect digestion or other derangement of the system, and in some persons and families, it may almost be said to be constitutional.

Treatment.—Persons subject to this affection cannot be too careful in keeping the teeth clean and free from tartar, and rinsing the mouth after every meal. With regard to medicines, the Specific No. Ten, two pellets morning and night, will correct it if dependent upon imperfect digestion. If it occurs in females during the monthly period, the Specific No. Eleven, two pellets morning and night, will remove the difficulty. Where it is constitutional or resists these medicines, the third trituration of *Aurum fol,* or of *Baryta carb.* a small powder taken daily, often works an entire cure.

## WANT OF APPETITE.

This may arise from various causes more or less intimately connected with the process of digestion, such as derangement of the stomach, inaction of the liver, results of over-eating, indigestion, etc. This morbid condition should be relieved in order that the natural desire for food should be manifested. When it seems to arise from a debilitated condition of the entire system, some stimulants, such as light wine or malt liquors may be taken with advantage. A glass of cold water taken morning and night is often beneficial in promoting an appetite. Aside from these measures, the Specific No. TEN, taken three times per day, two pellets before each meal, will generally be found efficacious.

## GASTRIC DERANGEMENT—INDIGESTION—BILIOUSNESS.

We distinguish this affection from chronic dyspepsia and from jaundice. It is very common and liable to come on suddenly, from irregularities in diet, over-eating, or partaking of heavy, rich, over-stimulating food, or food unsuited to the existing condition of the digestive organs; excessive use of wines, spirits, or strong malt liquors, or strong tea or coffee; eating too rapidly; irregularities in taking meals; too long fasting between meals; want of exercise; intense mental application; late hours, or from excesses of any kind. When the tone of the stomach has been weakened by purgatives, and in persons of naturally feeble digestion, this condition may be readily provoked by any transient violation of the ordinary regimen.

The symptoms are usually, want of appetite or deficient appetite; coated tongue; flat, insipid, putrid or bitter taste in the mouth; desire for acid, cooling or refreshing things;

frontal headache or heaviness of the head; dullness, stupidity or disposition to sleep; constipation, or sluggish, inactive bowels; and sometimes nausea, regurgitation of food, or vomiting of food and bile.

TREATMENT.—In general, little or no food should be taken into the stomach while the nausea and indisposition to food continues, only after these symptoms have passed away, should at first the more light and easily-digested food be given, such as water-gruel, rice-water, boiled rice, toast, or some nice ripe fruit. As medicine, the Specific No. TEN will be found sufficient, taken two pellets at a time, and repeated every three hours, until the condition has been removed.

Should there be fever, alternate the Specific No. ONE with No. TEN, at the intervals mentioned, and so continue until the febrile symptoms have yielded. Should there be nausea or vomiting, interpose between the portions of No. TEN, two or three doses of two pellets each of Specific No. SIX, until that symptom has been removed.

## CHRONIC DYSPEPSIA — INDIGESTION — WEAK STOMACH.

This is one of our most common diseases, and generally of very obstinate and lingering character. It may arise from various organic changes in the organs of digestion, and so may likewise manifest itself in diversified forms from the most trivial weakness of digestion, down to grave, organic changes in the substance of the stomach itself.

It may be induced or brought about by various causes, among which may be especially mentioned the use of cathartic or anodyne medicines in early life, or the habit of giving such drugs to infants; imperfect mastication of the food, in consequence of too rapid eating—a very common and wide-spread fault;—habitual low spirits and desponding state of mind, likewise weakens and impedes digestion; too long fasting, inducing exhaustion of the vital powers, likewise impairs the power of digestion; the excessive use of stimulants produces changes in the coat of the stomach which may render digestion difficult and finally impossible; want of exercise, sedentary habits, intense and long-continued mental application may likewise be named among its causes.

It is usually manifested by distress after eating; heaviness or weight in the pit of the stomach, as if a load or a stone lay there; tenderness of the præcordia on pressure; inability to wear tight clothes; frequent headache; dullness and confusion of the head; bloating after eating; sometimes water-brash, or rising of the food and fluid into the mouth after eating; want of appetite; bad taste; coated tongue; flatulence; constipation or sluggish or torpid bowels, and not unfrequently, piles or hemorrhoids. Such are among the more prominent symptoms by which this affection is manifested, yet they are constantly varied, relieved or intensified by the habits or food and regimen of the patient, or the intensity of the morbid condition.

Treatment.—The course usually pursued by the subjects of this disease tends much to aggravate and prolong it. Because the bowels are constipated, recourse is had to cathartic or aperient medicines, which afford only momentary relief, while permanently intensifying the disease. Costiveness may be bad, but not half so bad as the effects of drugs given to remove it. Persons subject to this disease should be careful of their diet. Use only such food as experience has taught them agrees with their digestion. A physician can only recommend the articles most likely to suit, and having ascertained from experience what diet or kinds of food are for the time best, the diet should be composed of these articles, and only by degrees as the digestion is improved, a more liberal bill of fare, or more questionable articles may be allowed. Take plenty of time for meals, eat moderately, and masticate the food well, using only a small quantity of fluid with the meal, and eat not too often, or too much at a time. Each night, on retiring, and in the morning on rising, take also a glass of cold water. Of medicines, the Specific No. TEN will usually be found efficient, and may be taken, two pills at a time, before each meal, and on retiring to rest at night. Perseverance in this course will rarely fail to cure the most inveterate and stubborn cases. If the bowels remain obstinately costive, an injection of tepid water may be taken every morning so long as it may be necessary. Very soon, under the influence of the medicine and proper food and habits, the bowels will act regularly.

## WATERBRASH—HEARTBURN.

These are merely symptoms of dyspepsia, or of gastric derangement. Yet, they may either of them form the principal feature of the complaint, and almost exclusively occupy the attention of the patient. In waterbrash there is a frequent rising or regurgitation of food or water more or less changed into the mouth from the stomach. Sometimes this is accompanied with belching of air coming up with the eructation, and accompanied with loud, unpleasant noise, and not unfrequently a large portion of every meal is thus thrown off. There is also a feeling of fullness, distention, and often of pain and distress in the stomach and præcordia.

With heartburn, there is a burning or gnawing uneasiness, felt principally in the pit of the stomach, but often extending far around or up into the chest, and down into the abdomen. Sometimes it is attended with anxiety, nausea, coldness of the extremities, debility and fever, faintness, and there are also sour, acrid risings, or regurgitations into the mouth.

TREATMENT.—As these are but symptoms or phases of dyspepsia or gastric derangement, the same treatment is indicated for both. Care in the selection and eating of food, and avoidance of the causes of indigestion, are important for a cure. As to medicine, the Specific No. TEN, two pills before each meal, and on retiring at night, or even morning and at night, will in general be found efficient. With females and delicate subjects the Specific No. ELEVEN may be equally or even more efficient, or the two may be taken in alternation.

## GASTRALGIA—PAIN OR SPASM OF THE STOMACH.

This is a very painful and distressing affection of the stomach, arising in most subjects of it, at somewhat regular periods of a few weeks or months, leaving the system in the interval comparatively free. It consists in spasmodic pains or contractions of the stomach, sometimes slight, but more commonly with almost insupportable violence; returning at intervals of a few moments with increasing vigor, after a comparative calm; the pain is most severe in the pit of the stomach, but often extends up into the chest and sides, or into the back, exciting nausea, vomiting and great anguish. Belching up of wind, which sometimes relieves the patient; faintness, coldness of the extremities, and anxiety are generally present. An attack may last from a few hours to one or two days, and it may return in some subjects at any time from very slight provocation, or at intervals of a few weeks or months, from no apparent cause.

The disease originates in a morbid condition of the nerves of the stomach, and is often associated with disease of the liver or spleen, or both, or in cancerous or other disorganizations of the stomach or intestines. An attack may be excited by eating indigestible food, fresh bread, chestnuts, sweetmeats, unripe fruit, cherries, figs, cheese, and in some cases, by taking coffee or strong tea. It may likewise, in gouty or rheumatic constitutions, be excited by exposure to cold and wet. In females it is sometimes found in connection with the monthly periods. In many instances the system seems to have acquired a predisposition to this form of disease, and in such subjects it masks or overshadows all other symptoms, and may be produced at any time from very slight indiscretions.

TREATMENT.—As precautionary measures, persons subject to this form of disease should be exceedingly careful in regard to their diet, avoiding rich food, gravies, fresh bread, warm cakes, preserves and cheese, or any article of food which experience has shown to disagree, or to occasion these attacks, and also to take as preventives, two pellets of the Specific No. TEN, morning and night. When any of the premonitory symptoms, or any slight gastric derangement threatens to culminate in an attack, recourse should be had at once to the Specific No. TEN, one or more doses of which, at intervals of two or three hours, will suffice to correct the derangement, and thus prevent the attack. During the attack, the Specific No. TEN is the proper remedy, and may be given in doses of two pellets, dissolved in a spoonful of water, and repeated every fifteen, thirty or sixty minutes, according to circumstances, until the pain is relieved. If the suffering is intense, and the pain not yield to the No. TEN, after an hour or so, it may be best to alternate the No. ONE in the same manner with it, and so continue until the patient is relieved. Hot cloths laid upon the stomach, and an injection of a large quantity of tepid water, are useful auxiliaries for relief during an attack.

## COLIC—BILIOUS COLIC.

Most persons are acquainted with what is termed bilious colic, though the disease is only occasionally caused by biliary derangements. It consists of paroxysms of greater or less degree of pain, generally very severe, felt more particularly about the navel, and thence extending upward or out over the abdomen. The pain is sharp, griping, tearing, cutting, or gnawing, coming on in paroxysms lasting a few moments and then remitting; sometimes the abdomen is drawn in, and at other times distended like a drum; pressure generally relieves the pain in colic, while in inflammation the pain is similar, while the abdomen is very sensitive and cannot be pressed upon, and in severe cases, cannot bear the slightest pressure. Sometimes the pains are accompanied by costiveness, and often by vomiting or diarrhœa. In colic there is seldom fever or heat of the surface, or a quick pulse, or pain on pressure, all of which are characteristic of inflammation. It may also be distinguished from hernia or rupture by the tumor either in the navel region or in the groin, which is always present and easily recognized in hernia.

Colic may be caused by excess in diet; flatulent food; dissipation; grief; cold, or anything that induces derangement of the digestive organs, or constipation of the bowels. Sometimes it arises from stricture of the intestine, or may in rare cases arise from cancerous disorganization of some portion of the intestine, or from *intussusception.*

*Flatulent, or wind colic,* is common in children who are fed with improper diet, and in dyspeptics after the use of heavy, improper or flatulent food.

*Bilious colic* is generally preceded by symptoms of biliary or gastric derangement, such as: Yellow-coated tongue, bitter taste, loss of appetite, dull headache. There is generally nausea and vomiting; severe, cutting, writhing pain, with thirst and anxiety; pain more especially extending from above the umbilicus towards the liver; coming on in severe, intense paroxysms. The pain is relieved after vomiting and discharge of free, bilious stools.

*Lead colic or Painters' colic* is produced by the exposure to the action of lead, and is common among painters who use white lead in their work, and among workers in lead-factories, or in smelting ores. The symptoms are: Loss of appetite, restless sleep, and nervous excitability. This is succeeded by vomiting, pain in the abdomen, coming on at first in paroxysms, but gradually becoming continuous. There is but little fever, but headache, pain in the limbs, and obstinate constipation, and sometimes even paralysis of the extremities. A bluish line along the edge of the gums may be often noticed in persons suffering from lead colic.

TREATMENT.—In general, and for ordinary attacks of colic, the Specific No. FIVE is the proper remedy, and will be found efficient. Should, however, the disease have been caused by heavy or indigestible food, or be accompanied with symptoms of gastric derangement, such as a coated tongue, bad taste, flatulence, etc., it will be well to alternate the Specific No. TEN with the No. FIVE. Dissolve twelve pellets of each Specific, in six large spoons of water, in separate glasses, and of these give alternately, every fourth or half hour, until relieved. This is the mode of procedure in all severe cases of colic from whatever cause, except that in cases where the bowels become tender, or sensitive on pressure, or there may be some fever, showing a tendency to the development of inflammatory action. In these latter cases, the Specific No. ONE should be prepared and given in alternation with No. FIVE, in the manner indicated above. Simple, uncomplicated spasmodic colic, yields promptly to the Specific No. FIVE, administered in water, two pellets every fifteen or twenty minutes.

In all cases of severe colic it is advisable, and in all obstinate cases, it may be necessary to administer to the patient, and the more so if caused by indigestible or noxious substances, INJECTIONS OF WARM WATER. To a pint of warm water, add a table-spoonful of salt, and with a good syringe, pump it into the abdomen. If the patient can retain it a little time, it may be more effectual, and these injections should be repeated until, in connection with the medicines, relief is obtained.

DIET.—It is obvious that little or no food, and that only of the lightest kind, such as oat-meal gruel, rice-water, toast-water, or some light soup, should be given until after the disease has yielded.

Persons subject to attacks of colic should be specially careful in avoiding the occasioning causes of it, such as indigestible food, the use of beans, cabbage, krout, or green vegetables, acidulated drinks, or veal or young meat; and should also be careful to keep the feet and abdomen dry and warm.

The use of the No. TEN Specific, two pellets at night, will also do much to correct the digestion, and so prevent attacks.

## NAUSEA AND VOMITING.

Nausea and vomiting seldom occurs except as a symptom of some other complaint or disease. If, as is frequently the case, it has been caused by over-loading the stomach, or the use of rich or indigestible food, or of noxious substances, it is clear that the effort of the system to rid itself of a hurtful substance by vomiting, should rather be promoted than arrested. Hence, in such cases, let the patient drink largely of warm water, or even titillate the throat with a feather or the finger, to promote the vomiting. After the noxious substance has been ejected, the Specific No. SIX, two pellets dissolved in a spoonful of water ana given every hour, will soon allay the remaining irritation, and relieve the nausea. When it occurs in the case of pregnant females, consult what is said under that head.

## SEA SICKNESS—SICKNESS FROM CAR OR CARRIAGE RIDING.

The peculiar sickness and utter wretcheaness and prostration experienced by persons on first going to sea, and even in a measure by some persons from riding in a car, stage, or wagon, is so well known as not to require description.

It can, however, in most cases, be cured by the Specific taken as follows:

Previous to sailing, the Specific No. TWENTY-SIX should be taken, if convenient, two pellets every four hours, permitting them to dissolve on the tongue.

After sailing, for the first two or three days, as a preventive, take two pills every four hours; and should there, notwithstanding, be severe sickness, vertigo, nausea, or vomiting, dissolve six or eight pills in half a glass of water, and take a dessert-spoonful every hour until relieved.

For sickness, nausea, or vomiting from riding in a carriage or similar motion, take of No. TWENTY-SIX, two of the pills, every hour until relieved.

## HEMATEMESIS—VOMITING OF BLOOD.

This disease is known by the vomiting, or sudden ejection of blood from the stomach. It is generally dark, rarely bright red, and is occasionally mixed with the food, mucus, bile, or other contents of the stomach, and is frequently thrown off in large quantities; blood is also frequently discharged by stool, in coagula. It may be known from bleeding of the lungs, by the absence of the cough or hehming which attends pulmonary hemorrhage; by the blood being generally darker, and by being thrown up by vomiting or retching, rather than by coughing. Vomiting of blood is always preceded by more or less decided symptoms of gastric disturbance or weak digestion, such as: Pressure, weight, fulness, or tensive pain in the region of the stomach; burning heat in that region; anxiety or uneasiness on partaking of food or drink, or on pressure of the stomach; saltish taste in the mouth; impaired appetite and nausea; vertigo, faintness, or cold perspiration; sometimes, also, an intermittent pulse is felt at the pit of the stomach. If the attack is very severe, there may be delirium or wandering of the mind, accompanied with spasms, and gradually increasing weakness and remission of pulse, with frequent fainting. It is most frequently caused by the suppression of some habitual discharge, as from hemorrhoids or the menstrual flow. Other causes, such as schirrhus, or internal lesions, or disorganizations of the stomach, or the use of poisonous or drastic purgatives, or an external contusion, or obstruction of some important viscera, may occasion congestion and the rupture of some vessels distributed over the surface of the stomach, and hence, become the immediate cause of the hemorrhage.

TREATMENT.—The first thing to do is to arrest the hemorrhage, and for this purpose HUMPHREYS' WITCH HAZEL is the most efficient remedy known, and may be given in doses of twenty drops, in a large spoonful of cold water, and repeated every fifteen or twenty minutes, until the bleeding is arrested, when it may be continued at intervals of an hour, or even a longer period, especially if the system seems exhausted, or there are yet indications of internal hemorrhage.

If there is fever or heat of the system, administer the Specific No. ONE, two pellets in a spoonful of water, and repeat every half hour. If it has come on in consequence of the suppression or non-appearance of the menstrual flux, the Specific No. ELEVEN should be given every hour, either alone or in alternation with the WITCH HAZEL. The diet should be carefully considered; all solid food must be avoided, and all warm drinks; animal jellies, preparations of milk, light puddings and broths, merely tepid, may be allowed in cases where the condition of the patient requires some nourishment, but no more food must be taken than is absolutely necessary to sustain the strength, and for some hours after an attack, no food should be given, and then, only in small quantities, and very cautiously.

## CHOLERA MORBUS.

This disease is of frequent occurrence in warm climates, and during the warm seasons of the year. It is generally brought on by the use of unripe fruit, or that which is over ripe, or stale, such as melons or cucumbers; or eating too much, or too many, or incongruous things at a time, and being over-heated afterwards; sudden changes of temperature; over-fatigue, or too free use of ice or ice-water.

The symptoms are violent vomiting and purging; throwing off the contents of the stomach and bowels at first, and afterwards bile; pain in the stomach and abdomen; thirst, and in severe cases, cramps, and coldness of the extremities; the face may also become pale, cold, bluish and sunken; features pinched, and cold, clammy skin, and great anxiety and prostration, similating an attack of cholera.

It is generally preceded by some symptoms indicating disturbance of the system, such as shivering, pain in the stomach and nausea, but in some cases it makes its attack without sensible premonitions.

It is liable to come on suddenly at night, and, properly managed, is of short duration.

TREATMENT.—The Specific No. SIX is the proper remedy, and may be administered by dissolving twelve pellets in six dessert-spoonfuls of cold water, of which a spoonful may be given every fifteen minutes, until the discharges are arrested and the warmth returned to the surface. In extreme cases, with violent cramps, coldness and blueness of the surface and great anguish, with little or no discharges, a dose of two or three drops of spirits of camphor, in a teaspoonful of water, repeated every few minutes, will soon relieve. The Specific, however, will be found promptly to arrest the disease. Diet should be light for some days, until the tone of the stomach is measurably restored.

## CHOLERA—ASIATIC CHOLERA.

As this terrible scourge is liable at any time to visit our country, and as the earlier treatment of it must frequently be entrusted to the hands of the people, it is most important that all should be acquainted with its earlier stages, and be prepared to meet them. Here we give the symptoms and treatment at greater length than may be required in other less important or sudden diseases.

PRECURSORS.—It has been frequently observed that the cholera has been preceded by some form of influenza, attended with sneezing, discharge from the eyes and nose, hoarseness, sore throat, and cough.

It has also been observed that previous to the outbreak of cholera in a particular locality, bowel complaints, as they are called, diarrhœa, dysenteries, colics, etc., have been much more frequent and obstinate, and less under the control of the ordinary remedies than usual, so that physicians, from these manifestations among their patients, have been able to recognize the presence of the disease in the atmosphere weeks before its final outbreak among the people.

Sudden attacks of cholera are more liable to occur at night and after midnight than during the day. Hence the necessity of every family being provided with prompt and efficient remedies to avoid the hurry, alarm and delay in sending for a physician in the night.

SYMPTOMS.—CHOLERA DIARRHŒA.—Almost invariably an attack of cholera is preceded by a peculiar form of diarrhœa. It may precede the cholera several days, as nothing more than loose bowels, attended with rumbling or borborigmi and slight nausea, or faintish feeling at the stomach, but usually it continues but a few hours, and is manifested with *frequent loose stools, rumbling and uneasiness* of the abdomen, and a *faintish, sinking sensation* at the pit of the stomach. This is the cholerine or cholera-diarrhœa, and the immediate precursor or first stage of the disease, and demands prompt attention.

After the diarrhœa has continued for a period varying from a few hours to several days, the second stage of the disease is ushered in with the following manifestations: REPEATED EVACUATIONS, attended with great prostration, at first, of the usual contents of the intestinal track, then gradually becoming more thin, watery and flocculent, until they present the true cholera characteristic of PROFUSE RICE WATER EVACUATIONS; vomiting in sudden, violent attacks, with copious discharges, first of the contents of the stomach, then of thin serum or the characteristic rice-water-like matter; attended with frequent cramps, first in the fingers, toes, and calves of the legs, then over the entire person, especially the abdomen, knotting up the limbs, and causing exquisite anguish. The breath becomes cold, the lips and tongue cold, the skin dry, inelastic, pale or leaden-gray, or a bluish-violet around the eyes and at the ends of the fingers and toes, and point of the nose, the hands becoming shrivelled like a washer-woman's. The face becomes peculiar in extreme cases, eye-balls glazed and turned up, pupils dilated, the upper eyelid drooping, the lower surrounded by a bluish half-moon; the color is pale, varying from a leaden gray to violet; the skin on the lips, cheeks, and point of the nose is glazed, nose pointed, cheeks sunken, upper lip drawn upward, the nostrils and cartilage of the ear very movable and wrinkled from the nose to the corners of the mouth, presenting a frightful and ghost-like appearance. The thirst is violent, less at first, but becoming inextinguishable during the progress of the disease. The voice becomes hoarse, whispering, or lost. The pulse at the wrist is very soft, small and disappearing during an attack of spasms, and later becomes thread-like and imperceptible. Gradually the anguish and indifference, the coldness and blueness, and prostration become more decided, until the patient sinks into a condition of absolute collapse, succeeded by death after some hours. During the attack, the secretion of the urine, the bile, the saliva, perspiration, and even of the tears, is entirely suppressed, and the reappearance of these secretions is a most favorable indication. With these manifestations of coldness, blueness, and shrivelled skin, and even cold breath, the patients yet complain of burning heat, long for ice and ice-water, and dread all heating applications.

Not always does the cholera present the above picture. Different epidemics have presented varieties in the symptoms which are very decided. Thus the disease has been divided into three stages, called the PREMONITORY, the stage of COLLAPSE and the stage of CONSECUTIVE FEVER.

The first, or PREMONITORY stage, is manifested by symptoms of indigestion, flatulence, weight or oppression at the pit of the stomach, slight nausea, acidity, diarrhœa, vertigo, some form of headache, or ringing in the ears. These symptoms may continue some time, occasionally pass off altogether, and leaving the patient well, but this is rare; and unless proper remedies are used, the symptoms above mentioned continue to increase until the second stage is ushered in.

SECOND STAGE—STAGE OF COLLAPSE—The stools at first feculent and bilious, now become characteristic; they appear like thin gruel or rice-water; sometimes they are limpid, intermixed with small flakes of curdy-looking matter; at others they look like water in which fresh beef has been macerated; sometimes the stools are even darker, looking like the dregs of wine. There is no natural smell from the stools, but a faint, peculiar odor, which also arises from the body. The desire to go to stool is irresistible and instantaneous, and sometimes with great tenesmus, accompanied by griping. Generally the stools are very copious—sometimes, however, they are scanty, often accompanied with discharge of noisy flatus from the bowels. There is *burning heat* in the pit of the stomach, and vomiting of large quantities of similar matter as the stools. The thirst is intense, with urgent desire for cold water. The mind generally remains clear, or comparatively so, but the vertigo and ringing in the ears increases. Cramps are almost universal attendants—sometimes confined to the fingers and toes; at others, affecting the legs and arms, and often the body, particularly the abdomen. The urine is generally suppressed; the voice is whispering. The respiration, though weak, is often natural, even when the pulse is scarcely perceptible at the wrist; occasionally, however, the breathing is hurried, oppressed, laborious. The pulse becomes weak and rapid early in the disease, even when the action of the heart is strong and tumultuous; but, frequently, both the pulse and heart are feeble. As the disease progresses, both become fainter and weaker; the pulse is only now and then felt like a "flutter," and often ceases at the wrist some hours before death. The tongue is cold and shrunk. The restless tossing, uneasiness, and impatience of the patient is pitiful; especially, when they are restrained, or when heat is applied, of which they seem to have a horror. The temperature of the body, especially of the extremities, diminishes early in the disease, and constantly sinks, until after death, when it gives place, for a time, to a genial warmth. As the disease progresses, the hands, feet, nails, face, and even the entire surface of the body, becomes ashen, leaden-gray, or blue, and this color remains or deepens until reaction occurs. Blood drawn from a vein or artery during this stage is of dark color, flows with difficulty, and does not coagulate. The surface of the body is covered with a cold moisture, the features and eye-balls shrunk, and death closes the scene—sometimes very unexpectedly, and at others, the body seems to be long dead, while the functions of the brain are still going on, and comparatively entire. In some cases the prostration of strength is great, but in others not so apparent.

Symptoms of improvement and recovery from the second stage are usually: Diminution of the number and quantity of the evacuations, both by vomiting and stools; cessation of the restlessness and tossing about; diminution of the cramps and thirst; increase of the strength and fullness of the pulse, and increase of the temperature of the body; more natural and animated expression of the countenance, and disposition to sleep; later, change of the stools from the watery to bilious and feculent matter; reappearance of the secretion of the urine. When these symptoms are manifested, they indicate the safety and early convalescence of the patient.

Consecutive stage.—In some rare cases, and in some epidemics more than others, patients instead of rallying at once from the second stage, slide over into what has been termed a third stage, or a typhus cholera, coming on after this fashion: The reaction has been established and patients seem to be doing well, not having tenesmus or vomiting, nor cramps, or any unusual degree of thirst, and the restlessness has passed off, and the patient seems to be tranquil. But gradually, symptoms of coma, deep sleep, or delirium come on, and there may be convulsions, partial paralysis, rigidity of the flexor muscles of the extremities, distressing nausea, bilious vomiting and thirst, difficult breathing or hurried respiration, cough, expectoration, palpitation or irregular action of the heart, more or less heat of the surface, bilious diarrhœa, dark port-wine, stools, tenesmus and pain or tenderness increased on pressure in some part of the abdomen. These symptoms may be variously combined and modified in particular cases, and may continue from four or five to fifteen days, ending in death, or the gradual recovery of the patient.

Hygienic Precautions to be observed during the presence of the Cholera.—All experience has demonstrated that the disease riots among the filthy, ill-fed, ill-clad, and ill-housed multitude; that its especial play-ground is along narrow streets, confined areas, ill-ventilated dwellings, low, damp, or confined apartments, and that the miasm is much more intense and concentrated in such localities than elsewhere, and its attacks far more intense and fatal. Hence, cleanliness, both of persons and habitations, is of the first importance.

The yard, gutter and cess-pool, should be cleansed often, and kept clean, and frequently sprinkled with chloride of lime, or plenty of lime, and the adjoining walls should be repeatedly whitewashed.

No stagnant water should be permitted in the cellar or yard, and if the basement is damp, fires should be kindled daily to expel foul air, and afford better ventilation.

All garbage should be removed daily, and nothing suffered to remain on the premises to be decomposed.

Houses should be daily ventilated.

Avoid damp, low habitations, and in selecting a residence, the higher and more airy the situation the better.

Narrow lanes and alleys, cellars and basements, and crowded apartments should be especially avoided.

The USUAL HABITS of eating, drinking, living, and business, should be followed, except when absolutely interdicted. Rash changes should be avoided.

Temperance in eating and drinking, exercise and labor, both physical and mental, is specially enjoined. Keep good hours.

Take proper food in reasonable quantities, at proper times.

Plainly cooked meats, lamb, beef, mutton, or fowl, with boiled rice or hominy, stale bread or crackers, and well-cooked potatoes, should form the ordinary staple of diet.

If wine or spirits are habitually used, they may be continued in moderation, but to persons not accustomed to them, they are especially objectionable and to be avoided. Drunkenness or debauchery powerfully invite the disease.

Avoid any kind of food or medicine which tends to relax the bowels.

Abstain from all unripe fruits, or stale, wilted, or over-kept vegetables.

Fruit of any kind should be avoided, if it induces loose bowels.

Cucumbers, salads, lettuce, cabbage, or krouts, soda-water, root-beer, melons, turnips, or unripe potatoes, are articles especially to be avoided.

Beer, cider, mineral-waters, are objectionable.

Purgative or cathartic medicines, by relaxing the integrity of the intestinal canal, may give rise to a sudden and fearful attack of the disease.

Avoid exposure and sudden changes of temperature, and at all times keep the body sufficiently warm and protected, especially the abdomen. To this end wear flannel next the skin, at least around the abdomen. Keep the feet and legs well protected and warm.

Above all things, maintain an even, cheerful tone of mind. Hurry, fright, fear, anxiety, and all depressing emotions, tend to lower the vital powers, and so invite the disease, while a firm determination to do our duty, and a cheerful reliance upon our Heavenly Father, are among the best safeguards.

PREDISPOSING CAUSES.—Persons of middle age are more subject to attack than infancy and old age. The female sex are considered more liable to it than males. Chronic diarrhœa predisposes the system for it, as do all prostrating or debilitating habits or excesses, scrofulous diathesis, and intermitting fevers. Among children, the male sex are more subject than the female sex, and those affected with sore mouth, jaundice, worms, and teething.

Infancy and old age are most exempt, and those suffering from ulcers of the legs, consumption, and influenza, least liable to an attatk.

PROPHYLACTICS.—*Preventive Treatment.*—The homely adage, "an ounce of prevention is better than a pound of cure," was never more clearly manifest than in this disease. Dirt, filth, irregular habits, and vice, induce the disease, while cleanliness, regularity, and order, keep it at bay. Aside from the hygienic observances enjoined above in regard to *living*, *labor*, and habits of thought, we earnestly reccommend, also, the use of a simple medicinal prophylactic or preventive. Experience has amply demonstrated the utility of medicinal prophylactics. It has abundantly shown that small-pox, scarlet-fever, measles, hooping-cough, and fevers, as well as cholera, can be prevented by fortifying the system by appropriate medicinal influences. Not, indeed, by drugging, overwhelming and thus depressing the system, but by the judicious use of the (similar) HOMEOPATHIC Specific, which, by pervading and preoccupying the system, fortifies it against, and thus prevents an attack of the disease. Hence, we advise the use of the Specific No. Six, in doses of two pellets, morning and at night, as a true prophylactic for the cholera. Safer still will it be to send for a case of the Cholera Specifics in fluid form, and to follow the directions there given.

Directions.—Live temperately, avoid the predisposing causes of the disease as before mentioned, avoid coffee and camphor, which might antidote the effects of the medicine, and take each morning, on rising, or before breakfast, and each night on retiring, two pellets of the Specific No. Six. Children need but one-half as much as adults. In families, the best manner is to place the proper number of pellets for each person in a glass, and add a large spoonful of water for adults, and a teaspoonful for children, and so give them, morning and night, while the disease prevails. Travelers may simply take the Specific dry on the tongue, if other conveniences are wanting. The result will be, that either no attack will occur, or it will be in a modified and very mild form.

Treatment of the Cholera Diarrhœa, *or Premonitory Stage of the Disease.*—The earlier symptoms of the disease are: A sense of uneasiness, or sinking at the pit of the stomach, rumbling, or borborigmi in the bowels, and loose stools or diarrhœa. Sometimes, to these symptoms are added, acidity of the stomach, griping pains in the abdomen, vertigo or headache, and ringing or noise in the head.

So soon as the above symptoms, or even the diarrhœa alone has declared itself, the patient should retire at once to his home, or room, and lie down, taking four pellets of the Specific No. Four. If the symptoms are only slight, that is, only some diarrhœa, and slight uneasiness of the bowels, repeat the dose every hour, or every two hours. But if the stools are urgent or frequent, with uneasiness and nausea, vertigo and sinking at the stomach, repeat the dose every half hour until relieved.

If the diarrhœa should not yield in, say four or six hours, under the influence of the Specific No. FOUR, administered as above directed, and the disease threatens to pass over into the second stage, indicated by more frequent or urgent stools, coldness, nausea, or some faintness at the pit of the stomach, then omit for a time the diarrhœa Specific, and give the Specific No. SIX, repeated every half hour, in its place. In rare cases the CAMPHOR has been efficient in checking the diarrhœa, in doses of two drops of the tincture on a bit of sugar, every half hour.

Rarely will more than two or three doses of the Specific be required to check and control the disease at this stage, provided, also, that the following conditions are observed:

IT IS OF THE UTMOST IMPORTANCE that the patient should lie down in bed, get warm, keep well covered, with a bottle of hot-water, or hot bricks, to the feet, if necessary, and so remain warm and in bed, until the diarrhœa, rumbling and uneasiness has passed off. Being about, or frequently getting up, and running out, is very prejudicial, and most surely tends to prolong and keep up the disease.

AVOID TREPIDATION, OR HURRY, unnecessary anxiety, or alarm in prescribing for yourself or others. Do not multiply doses, or measures of relief, from which nothing is permitted to avail, but give every dose carefully, and then give it time to act, and afford relief, and only when one has failed, give another. The one course perseveringly followed will be successful, while if you attempt others, all will fail. Nothing but Homeopathic medicines must be given under Homeopathic treatment. All other medicines or means interfere and must not be allowed.

THIS STAGE MAY END in health: By the stools becoming less frequent and finally natural, the rumbling, uneasiness of the bowels disappearing, and the sinking or anxiety at the præcordia going off, or:—it may terminate in the next stage by the stools becoming more frequent and fluid, the uneasiness and sinking increasing, until vomiting comes on with the characteristics of the second stage.

TREATMENT OF THE CHOLERA PROPER, *or Second Stage of the Disease.*—This stage is known by profuse, thin, flocculent, or rice-water-like evacuations coming on suddenly and frequently. Sudden vomiting of the same or similar material, attended with cramps in the extremities, or even body, and great coldness or blueness of the surface, anxiety and prostration, and other symptoms, as before described.

Where this condition, PROFUSE VOMITING AND DIARRHŒA, is present, the Specific No. SIX is only required, of which give five pellets, either at once upon the tongue, or better, in a spoonful of cold or ice-water, and repeat the dose, EVERY FIFTEEN OR TWENTY MINUTES, according to the result, and so continue until the cramps, the vomiting and diarrhœa have abated, when the intervals between the doses may be prolonged to half an hour, and then, gradually, as the patient improves, to intervals of an hour or more.

THE PATIENT SHOULD AT ONCE go to bed, and, if possible, not get up to attend to the evacuations, but use a bed-pan, or other convenience, for that purpose. Bottles of hot water, or hot bricks, should be placed to the feet, if the patient can bear them. Give nothing but the medicine and small sips of ice-water; or better, give from time to time small pieces of ice, to remain in the mouth to allay the thirst. These are better than water or other fluid, more grateful, and less likely to provoke vomiting, stools or griping. Let the patient remain quiet as possible after the storm is over, and if he falls asleep, do not waken him, even to administer medicine.

TO ALLAY THE CRAMPS, it is better to grasp and hold the knotted limb or part in the warm, firm hand, than merely to rub the surface, as you may, by severe rubbing, easily excoriate the surface, without relieving the cramp, while the warm pressure of the hand is very grateful and effective.

IF THE ATTACK occurs in the following form from the first, or if in the course of the disease this condition is developed, viz.: but little, or only slight vomiting, or purging, or scanty evacuations, but great dullness or confusion of the head, severe, frequent, long-continued cramps, predominant coldness and blueness of the surface, loss of voice, and *weak, thread-like,* or *wanting pulse,* give at once five drops of SPIRITS OF CAMPHOR, in half a teaspoonful of cold water, and repeat the dose every ten minutes, or even every five minutes, in extreme cases, until the returning pulse, or warmth of the surface, and returning evacuations show the reaction of the system to have come on. Then gradually omit the CAMPHOR, and return to the use of the Specific No. SIX, which continue every fifteen or thirty minutes, and at longer intervals, until entire relief is obtained. The camphor is the best remedy to arrest the *sinking, coldness, blueness, failing pulse,* and tendency to absolute collapse; and when the evacuations have ceased, or nearly so, a few doses, given at intervals of five or ten minutes, will promptly bring up the pulse and warmth to the surface, and with this reaction the vomiting and evacuations may again return. Then the Specific comes again in use and may be continued as above mentioned, a dose of five drops every ten or twenty minutes, until the evacuations have ceased and relief is fully pronounced.

AFTER THE STORM has passed over, and the vomiting, diarrhœa, and cramps have vanished, and returning pulse, warmth, sleep, and rest, and secretions have become re-established, a little nourishment may be given. This should consist of very light meat broth, and in very small quantities at first, as experience has shown that the stomach long remains weak after an attack, and heavy or indigestible food, or any food in too large quantity, may easily provoke a relapse, always more dangerous than the original attack. Hence, give at first a little weak black tea, or chicken or lamb broth; afterwards boiled rice, toasted bread, and only very gradually return to a more substantial diet.

The patient will remain weak and enfeebled for some time, and not unfrequently, the digestive organs are long in regaining their former strength and vigor. For this debility, beer and good malt liquor have proved beneficial. Too free perspiration diminishes the strength; and slight mental excitement, too much warmth, too much drink or food, cause anguish, palpitation, small, soft pulse, vomiting or diarrhœa, uneasy sleep, and extreme debility.

THE SECOND STAGE MAY TERMINATE in convalescence, indicated by: Diminished violence and frequency of the evacuations, first the vomiting, later the diarrhœa; diminution of the cramps; increasing strength and fullness of the pulse; returning warmth of the surface; more natural expression of the countenance; less tossing about, restlessness and jactitation; diminished thirst; bilious stools; natural warmth of the surface; return of the natural secretions, urine, saliva and perspiration; quiet, tranquil sleep; or, this condition may slide into the third stage indicated by the following symptoms :—

Diminished vomiting; great indifference; extreme prostration; the patient lying on the back, sinks down towards the foot of the bed; some return of warmth or moisture to the skin; increasing lividity or blueness of the surface, and the *blue, sunken, pointed* CHOLERA FACE; the pulse cannot be felt, and later, not even at the carotids or heart; eyes dull and glassy; only occasional and not characteristic vomiting and diarrhœa; later, the stools are involuntary, as if coming from a spout; respiration labored, rattling and almost ceasing. This stage may last from one or two hours, to as many days, and usually terminates in death, preceded by cold, clammy sweats, complete cessation of circulation and respiration, and final paralysis of the lungs.

TREATMENT.—In this stage of entire collapse, which may last a day or two, the patient is not absolutely hopeless, and should be carefully and judiciously treated. The case will doubtless be placed in the hands of a competent Homeopathic physician, who, by the alternate use of Carb. veg. and Arsenicum, administered every hour, may save the patient.

As the pulse comes up, the medicine may be given at longer intervals. It is useless, and often cruel, to make hot applications to the patient, who, however cold, complains of heat, and refuses all covering. Hence, make them comfortable, covering only as decency and the weather requires, give the medicines and patiently await the result. It will, oftentimes, be favorable, even in these worst cases.

☞I have prepared a case of three large ONE OUNCE VIALS of Specifics for the special treatment of CHOLERA, and in case of the prevalence of this disease, I recommend its use, as the Specifics are in fluid form, and in larger quantities and more reliable during an epidemic. If the case of Cholera Specifics is used, it is only necessary to substitute drops for pellets, or adopt the directions which come with the case.

## DIARRHŒA—LOOSENESS OF THE BOWELS.

We generally understand by this term a disease or condition in which the bowels are moved more frequently than in health, and the stools are more or less fluid in form. The stools may be very numerous, or be only two or three in the twenty-four hours, and may be of almost every variety of character and consistence. They are often greenish, yellowish, mixed or closed up, frothy, foamy, or serous, thin, watery, or at times bloody, though this is generally characteristic of dysentery. Usually the pain is trifling, but sometimes the pain, griping or aching in the bowels is quite severe.

Sometimes loose bowels or a transient diarrhœa is merely the salutary effort of the system to rid itself of some injurious or indigestible substance, and hence, when there is reason to suspect such a condition, it is proper to wait a reasonable period before attempting to arrest it, and only when the condition is clearly morbid, seek to control it by the proper means.

When the evacuations seem to afford the patient relief, it is safe to wait a day or so to see if it is not merely a salutary effort of nature, and which will speedily correct itself.

Diarrhœa may be induced by a cold, or a sudden check of perspiration, disordered stomach, use of improper food, fright, fear, vexation, or excessive heat.

The irritation of teething in children is one of the most frequent causes of diarrhœa, and it is generally observed that teething children who have diarrhœa, are less liable to serious illness than those who have constipated bowels.

Diarrhœa, also, usually comes on at the close of several diseases, as some forms of fever, measles and consumption.

Treatment.—The Specific No. Four is appropriate for almost all forms of diarrhœa and loose bowels, and will speedily control it. It may be given dry on the tongue, two pellets at a dose, and repeat at intervals of from an hour to two or three hours, according to the urgency of the case. Should the stools be loose, thin, watery, or urgent, and especially if there should be some nausea or vomiting, the Specific No. Six should be given in alternation with No. Four, as before directed. Should there be pain, griping, or straining, showing a tendency to dysentery, the Specific No. Five is appropriate, and may be given alone, or in alternation with the No. Four.

Diet and general management.—Rest and quiet are very beneficial in all severe cases of diarrhœa. The patient should avoid acids, coffee, and all highly seasoned, salted articles of food, also, all fruit, eggs, oysters, and chicken or veal. The diet should be: Stale bread, rice, hominy, oatmeal, barley, or drinks made from these. Milk, thickened with flour, or mutton-soup, thickened with rice or oatmeal. As the appetite returns, the diet may be more liberal, but still care and discretion should be exercised in the selection of food until the disease is arrested.

## CHRONIC DIARRHŒA.

This condition is quite common in the hot climates or where persons have been long exposed to the unfavorable influences of climate, exposure or bad food. It is often, also, the result of badly-cured fevers and diseases of the liver, and a not rare result of an imperfectly cured dysentery. It may also be the result of scrofulous disease of the bowels, tubercular deposits, or degeneration of the follicular and mucus surface, or of ulceration. The stools vary according to the seat, location, and character or nature of the local degeneration from which they arise. They are however, frequent, more or less liquid, sometimes mucopurulent, or may at times be even blood-stained or mucus. They are usually accompanied by general prostration, impaired digestion, emaciation, or other evidences of organic disease.

Treatment.—The alternate use of Specifics Nos. Four and Five have proved curative in numerous cases. Two pellets may be given at a time, dry on the tongue, and repeated every four hours, in alternation. For diet, consult what is said under diarrhœa.

## DYSENTERY.

Dysentery generally prevails in the late summer and fall of the year, when the days are hot and the nights cool. It is often epidemic, but may be induced by exposure to drafts of air, over-exertion, sitting on the damp or cold ground, use of acid or unripe fruits, or stale fruits and vegetables, melons, cucumbers, etc. It is liable to attack all ages and both sexes, but is more dangerous for infants, children, the aged, and females generally, than for men.

An attack of dysentery is usually preceded for some days, or in some cases only for a few hours, by precursory symptoms, such as: Sense of general depression, pains in the neck, back, or limbs, headache, loss of appetite, chilliness, heat, transient sweats, nausea or vomiting. Gradually there are colic pains passing about the bowels, in the navel region, and along the course of the colon; rumbling, and a feeling as if there was some foreign body low down in the rectum, producing an inclination to stool, and diarrhœa, or in some cases constipation.

The disease is characterized by pains in the abdomen, which pass from the navel region to the right, then up and across the abdomen and down the left side, and extending towards the rectum, terminate by producing the tenesmus or urgent desire for stool. Usually these pains and tenesmus precede every stool, and often remain quite a time after it, and so there may be an almost incessant urging to stool, caused by the swelling and irritation of the rectum. This feeling of tenesmus or straining, a violent constriction of the rectum, is a characteristic of the disease. The stools are peculiar, very frequent, often twelve, twenty-four, fifty, or more in the twenty-four hours. Sometimes the urgency is so constant that the patient can scarcely leave the vessel. The quantity is very small, often not more than a spoonful, and consists of mucus, fluid, or coagulated blood, more or less mixed with greenish or mucus masses, or membranous patches like scrapings of the intestines, with little or no fecal matter. Often there is fever, thirst, headache, hot, dry skin, accelerated pulse, diminished urine, sleeplessness, and the abdomen is painful to contact.

The disease may continue eight or ten days, and terminate in recovery by the remission of the colic and tenesmus, stools becoming less frequent, more copious and feculent, warm perspiration, quiet and sleep coming on; or it may end fatally, with increase of violent symptoms, until peritonitis, or a typhus condition sets in. Under our treatment it is rarely fatal, except in quite young children, and generally terminates in health in four or six days.

TREATMENT.—The Specific No. FIVE is the appropriate remedy, and may be administered, if the stools are quite frequent, as often as every twenty or thirty minutes, in doses of two pellets, dissolved in a small spoonful of water. Should there be considerable fever, thirst and restlessness, the Specific No. ONE may be given in alternation with No. FIVE at the same intervals until the fever is subdued, when the No. FIVE should be continued alone, at intervals of from half an hour, to one or two hours, diminishing the frequency of the doses as the disease is subdued.

DIET AND REGIMEN.—When the disease comes on, the patient should at once keep quiet; avoid exercise or labor of any kind; if possible, lie down, and confine himself strictly, during the whole course of the disease, to a porridge made of milk and flour well cooked, or to farina gruel, or rice-water and boiled rice. No vegetables or fruit can be allowed, nor meat, nor meat-broths; and spirits, or stimulants of any kind, are absolute poisons. Use no other medicines of any kind. Opium only conceals the disease by quieting the pain and evacuations, while the disease rages more destructively.

During the disease, if the evacuations are very frequent

and the tenesmus or straining very distressing and painful, occasional injections of thin starch may be given, or the patient may have a seat-bath of tepid water for a short time. This course strictly followed will rarely fail to afford decided relief in from twelve to twenty-four hours, and an entire cure in four or six days.

## CONSTIPATION—COSTIVE BOWELS.

This condition can scarcely be called a disease. It is mainly a symptom of some morbid condition of the system, upon the removal of which, this inconvenience is relieved. In many cases it is habitual, the stools are hard, dry and infrequent, which indeed often indicates a more healthy and vigorous condition of the system than a diarrhœa, or even soft, frequent stools. The philosophy of the condition itself is but little understood. The fecal matter is a secretion, and as this is eliminated, it passes into the common receptacle, the rectum, and there remaining until the irritation caused by its presence, or the evolutions of the system, occasion its expulsion in the form of feces. Whether this expulsion shall occur every twelve, twenty-four, forty-eight, or sixty hours, or six days, or as I have known in one case, fourteen or sixteen weeks, depends altogether upon circumstances. Though the fact of an undue or unnatural accumulation or retention, does not of itself constitute disease. It is an inconvenience, and may occasion disease, or may not, or may be occasioned by a morbid condition of the system. Whenever the morbid condition is relieved, the bowels will of themselves act naturally, and the retention will be avoided.

The difficulty itself is usually greatly aggravated by the means employed to cure it. Cathartic or aperient medicines may move the bowels for the time. But after the first operation is exhausted, the reaction of the system comes on, and the bowels are more constipated than before. Then new and larger doses, and stronger and more active medicines are used, until an almost incurable condition is induced. It should be remembered that cathartics are always injurious in cases of habitual constipation, the disease often originating in dryness and irritation of the lining of the intestinal track, the very condition which cathartics engender and sustain. It may be safely averred that no case of habitual constipation was ever cured by cathartic medicines, while thousands of cases have been aggravated or rendered incurable by them. In one condition the operation of a cathartic or laxative medicine is allowable. When some hurtful or indigestible substance has been taken into the system, which does not pass off, and by its presence causes irritation, fever, pain, convulsions or other inconvenience. In such cases, a spoonful of castor oil acts as a prompt laxative, and removes the offending substance without drugging or medicating the system, and is altogether the safest and most efficient remedy.

Treatment.—Persons subject to constipation will generally find some form of indigestion connected with it, and on the removal of this, the constipation will vanish. But they should, moreover, be careful in regard to diet; eat slowly, masticate the food sufficiently, choose relaxing articles of diet, fruits, wheaten grits, coarse bread, farina, puddings of rice, bread, and sauce of prunes, peaches, or plums. Use fresh beef, mutton, or lamb, and soups made of them, avoiding salted meats, cheese, rice, and bread or crackers made of superfine flour. Cold water should be used freely, and a glass drank on going to bed and on rising each morning, are important auxiliaries. At times, constipation has been induced and sustained by an insufficient degree of heat in the bowels, and this has been obviated, and a cure effected by wearing a *flannel swathing around the bowels.*

Lastly, the habit of going to stool every morning should be formed and persisted in; go regularly, and wait a certain time, if at first, fruitlessly. With these helps, and the use of the Specific No. TEN, two pellets dissolved in water and taken each morning and at night, the difficulty will soon be overcome, and regular, healthy evacuations established.

## PILES—HEMORRHOIDS.

This troublesome and frequently obstinate disease is very common. The symptoms are varied according to the character of the disease and the stage of its development. Most commonly there are discharges of blood from time to time from the anus, more frequently during a hard stool, but in severe cases the blood may be discharged at other times, and sometimes in quite large quantities, often attended with a feeling of relief. Tumors are frequently formed about the anus, or within the rectum, which come down or are protruded at every stool. They may be small, bluish, filbert or walnut size, or even much larger, single or grouped in clusters, sometimes painless, but often inflamed, painful and tender, and they may remain dry, or discharge, forming either mucus or bleeding piles. In some cases a violent itching and irritation within the rectum seems to be the predominant characteristic of the disease. During what is termed an attack of piles, the patient has a sense of fullness and heaviness of the abdomen, pain in the lower part of the back, fullness of the head or headache, failing appetite or indigestion, which is relieved often after a discharge of blood from the tumors.

The disease is always the result of abdominal venous congestion, from whence results engorgement of the hemorrhoidal veins, distributed over the rectum, the swelling of the mucous membrane, formation of tumors, and frequent discharge of blood.

It is more frequent among persons of sedentary habits, and much favored by the use of spirits, coffee, highly spiced and indigestible food, late hours and intense mental application. Some temperaments, the dry, meagre, bilious, are more subject to them than others; they are also quite common with pregnant and lying-in women.

It is common for old school treatment to excite these tumors in attempting a radical cure. But it will be seen that this is only disposing of the results of the disease, leaving the causes still at work, and the consequence is that the tumors form again, either at the same place, but more frequently higher up, and in a more difficult and inaccessible locality. Our treatment requires no such expedients, as we possess the means of reaching the disease at its source, and of permanently curing it.

TREATMENT.—Persons subject to piles, and those suffering from an attack of the disease, should not be altogether careless in regard to diet. A fit of indigestion often brings on an attack of piles; hence, use easily digested, relaxing food, use some care in the selection of food, and much care in properly masticating it. Graham bread, or that made of unbolted or coarse flour is beneficial, and so is the free use of wheaten grits, farina, and other relaxing food. For medicine, the Specific No. SEVENTEEN, two pellets, three times per day—morning, noon and night—for cases of chronic piles. If there is dyspepsia or indigestion also, the Specific No. TEN may be given in alternation with it, taking two pellets before each meal, and on going to rest at night. Should there be an attack of piles, the tumors becoming swelled, painful and tender, the Specifics No. ONE and No. SEVENTEEN should be given in alternation, each dissolved in water, two pellets in a large spoonful, and administered every one or two hours until relief is afforded, then go on with the No. SEVENTEEN for a permanent cure. Should there be bleeding or internal piles, the above will be proper and promptly efficient treatment.

For an external application the WITCH HAZEL diluted, one-half with water, and applied with a T bandage to the part, is the best possible remedy, and promptly allays the pain and inflammation. Its injection, when the tumors are internal, give very prompt relief, and in case of chronic bleeding piles, a large spoonful of the undiluted WITCH HAZEL, thrown into the rectum on retiring at night, will work like a charm. During a severe attack of piles, the patient should, as far as possible, maintain a recumbent position, and all chronic cases of piles will find an improvement to have the stool AT NIGHT in preference to the morning. If the bowels are costive, injections of water should be used freely, in order to have a daily movement.

## PROLAPSUS ANI—PROTRUSION OF THE INTESTINE.

This affection is not uncommon in children, and is occasionally met with in adults. It is generally the result of straining while at stool, in connection with a weakness or relaxed condition of the sphincter of the rectum. Sometimes the parts are protruded several inches, and in other cases but slightly, and readily return of themselves. When the protrusion does not return of itself, as is sometimes the case in children, the child should be laid upon its side, and the part gently pressed upon with the hand which has been oiled, or a cloth wet in cold water, or oil or soft lard, and the pressure continued gently until the reduction is effected.

To prevent a recurrence of the prolapsus, the Specific No. TEN, two pills at night, and the No. THIRTY-FIVE, two pills each morning, will be the proper remedies. The same treatment is proper for chronic tendency to prolapsus. If the prolapsus occurs in the course of diarrhœa, the cure of the diarrhœa will also arrest the tendency to prolapsus.

## LIVER COMPLAINT.

This disease may be divided into the acute and chronic forms, the latter, however, is generally known by the name of liver complaint, although a careful examination of the disease, will many times reveal the fact, that the real disease is rather in the stomach and bowels than the liver. In some cases the liver itself may have become implicated, and may become properly the subject of treatment. Consult *Chronic Inflammation of the Liver.*

## ACUTE INFLAMMATION OF THE LIVER—HEPATITIS.

This disease is more common in the Southern States of the Union and in the tropical climates, than in the Northern or Middle. In the Southern States, the use of fat and heavy food, exposures to heavy dews or damps in the evening, and the powerful rays of the sun by day, are among its most frequent exciting causes. It may also be caused by violent mental emotions, the use of stimulants or ardent spirits, suddenly suppressed evacuations, violent emetics or purgatives, the abuse of mercury, gall stones, external lesions, or even injury of the brain.

The symptoms differ according to the seat of the inflammation. When this attacks the outer or convex surface of the liver, the symptoms closely resemble those of pleurisy; there is usually a violent pain in the right hypochondrium or liver region, sometimes resembling stitches, at others burning, shooting to the breast-bone, the shoulder-blade, or the point of the shoulder, or the right limb; sensation of numbness or tingling in the arm of that side, the pain increased by inspiration; a dry, short cough, and symptoms of acute fever; bowels irregular, generally constipated, and stools in the majority of cases of an unnatural color. In this form, the patient can only lie on the left side. When the seat of the inflammation is upon the inner or concave surface of the liver, the pain is much less, and the patient complains rather of a sensation of pressure than of actual pain, but the entire biliary system is much more involved. The eyes and face become yellow, as in case of jaundice; the urine is orange-colored, the evacuations mostly hard, and generally of a whitish or clay color. We also find bitter taste in the mouth, vomiting and distress in the region of the liver. The patient can only lie on the right side. The fever is usually high also in this form.

Inflammation of the liver, unless properly treated, is liable to assume a chronic form, and may also terminate in suppuration, and the matter communicate with the lungs or the intestinal track; or may form a vomica or point and discharge externally; or it may form indurations or other alterations of structure in the liver, or result in the formation of adhesions.

TREATMENT.—The Specific No. ONE is the proper remedy from the first, and should be continued either alone or in alteration with some other Specific, until the disease is subdued. Dissolve twelve pellets in six spoonfuls of water, and of this give a large spoonful every hour for the first twenty-four or forty-eight hours, or until the fever is mostly subdued, and pain and distress relieved. Then prepare the Specific No. TEN in the same manner, and give the two medicines in alternation, at intervals of two or three hours, until the disease is subdued and convalescence established.

The diet should be the same as in fevers or other inflammations: toast-water, thin gruel of corn or oat-meal, milk-toast or light meat-soups, according to the stage of the disease.

## LIVER COMPLAINT—CHRONIC INFLAMMATION OF THE LIVER.

There are numerous morbid conditions of the liver which are popularly known as liver complaint, such as, enlargement, softening, abscesses, adhesion with adjacent organs, or the result of acute inflammation. What passes as dyspepsia, is often some morbid condition or degeneration of this organ.

The symptoms of chronic inflammation of the liver are essentially those of acute inflammation, with the distinction of their duration, and their being less clearly expressed, and their slower progress, and fever also only comes on after the disease has made considerable progress. The usual symptoms are as follows: Weight in the stomach after eating, flatulence, cramp of the stomach, acid eructations, nausea, sometimes bilious vomiting, loss of appetite or canine hunger, thirst, whitish dry tongue, bitter taste, feeling of heat, heaviness, fullness or dull pain in the region of the liver and epigastrium, and tenderness of these regions on pressure; sometimes the pain is wanting or comes at irregular intervals, or is increased by exercise or filling the stomach; often sympathetic pains in the right shoulder, wandering pains in the limbs, alternating with those in the liver region; feeling of numbness or of paralysis in the lower extremities. There is often distention of the liver region, protrusion of the liver down below the false ribs, especially in a sitting or upright position of the body; difficult lying on the left or on either side, constipation, feces hard, without bile, clay or putty like; sometimes diarrhœa, dark mixed-like tea-grounds, or flocculent stools; not unfrequently, vomiting of dark, adhesive, coagulated blood. The urine is thick, yellowish, oily, or scant, with thick sediment; often dry, hollow cough, with inability to take a deep inspiration; yellow or an earthly pale complexion, but in some cases there is not a trace of jaundice present. Usually there is mental depression and despondency, unquiet sleep or sleeplessness. In the latter stages the pulse, which up to this period had been slower than in the normal condition, becomes feverish towards evening. The disease often makes but slow progress, continuing for years, with frequent pauses at irregular intervals.

TREATMENT.—The Specific No. TEN is generally the best remedy, and may be taken in portions of two pellets, dry on the tongue, before each meal and on going to rest at night. Should there be at any time heat, fever or swelling, or tenderness of the region of the liver, the Specific No. ONE should be administered in fluid form, every two hours, as directed for acute inflammation of this organ. Aside from this, the use of Specific No. TEN should be relied upon for a permanent cure of this disease. Diet as for DYSPEPSIA.

## JAUNDICE.

This disease is well known, and may occur to persons at all ages of life. It may continue for weeks, or even months, and there are some who are quite subject to such attacks. The disease generally commences with some form of indigestion, such as: Loss of appetite, somnolence, constant drowsy, dull feeling, giddiness or swimming of the head, flatulence, nausea, vomiting, and there is some degree of tension or sense of pressure in the region of the liver. Gradually the face and skin, and especially the whites of the eyes, become yellow, and in some cases the skin becomes dark-brown, or even black, giving rise to the appellation of "black jaundice;" the urine becomes orange colored, and the feces whitish, clay, or putty-like, and there may be pain in the region of the liver. There is also frequently a very disagreeable tingling of the skin. It is likewise attended with more or less depression of spirits and loss of strength. In general there is but little fever, but in severe cases there may be an unusual amount of fever, with a tendency to the brain, producing a sort of stupid sleep, from which the patient is aroused with difficulty. This condition may be considered dangerous, as a fatal result may follow from oppression of the cerebral organs. When the disease has been caused from some unusual mental emotion, it may come on very suddenly, but in general it comes on in a very gradual, and not unfrequently, unobserved manner. It may be caused by acute or chronic inflammation of the liver; or from diseases of the stomach, or other portions of the intestinal track; blows upon the head, or in the region of the liver, may produce the disease; also moral emotions, or violent fits of passion; the inordinate use of quinine, rhubarb or calomel, or other forms of mercury, may also be mentioned as causes, as these agents often tend to obstruct the biliary duct.

TREATMENT.—The Specifics No. ONE and No. TEN are the proper remedies. In slight cases, two pellets of No. ONE each morning, and two more pellets of No. TEN at noon and night will be sufficient. Should the disease be more decided and well marked, and the patient have some degree of fever, the two remedies mentioned may be taken in alternation, two pellets every two hours until amendment occurs, and then at somewhat longer intervals until the disease is cured.

The diet should be of easily-digested food, free from condiments or stimulants of any kind, and may consist chiefly of chicken or veal soup, with stale bread, tapioca, sago or rice, and gruels made of arrow-root, corn-starch or farina. The drink should be principally water, and all stimulating or tonic bitters made of cider, barks, or wine, should be avoided, and especially all indigestible food, such as eggs, butter, fat-meats, milk, etc.

# DISEASES OF THE URINARY AND GENITAL ORGANS.

## INFLAMMATION OF THE KIDNEYS.

This disease is known by a pungent aching pain in the small of the back, on one side, generally the left, alongside of the spine, in the region of the kidneys. The pain is constant, and but slightly increased by contact or pressure, extending forward and downward along the course of the ureter. The secretion of urine is diminished when only one kidney is affected, and even entirely arrested in those rare cases where both are involved. There is frequent urging to urination, pain in the urethra, especially at the neck of the bladder during urination, sometimes even cramps of the bladder, and hence difficulty in voiding it. The urine is dark red, and often shows traces of blood. Not unfrequently the bladder becomes involved, and occasions a permanent constrictive pain in that region, which is increased by contact or pressure over the part. There is likewise nausea or even actual vomiting, sharp, decided fever, usually commencing with a severe chill, followed by heat; dry, hot skin, coated tongue, extreme thirst, full, hard, tensive pulse.

The disease is rather rare, but it may arise in consequence of gout, or renal calculi, or be occasioned by a fall, or injury in the kidney region; or by suppression of the hemorrhoidal or menstrual flow, or by the use of certain medicines, such as squills, cantharides, etc.

TREATMENT.—If there is considerable fever, the treatment may commence with the Specific No. ONE, of which two pellets may be dissolved in water and given every half-hour for three or four hours. Then the Specific No. THIRTY may be given in alternation with it at the same intervals. Dissolve twelve pellets of each in six spoonfuls of water, each of No. ONE and No. THIRTY, in separate glasses, and of these give every hour a spoonful in alternation, until the fever has abated, then substitute the No. TWENTY-SEVEN for the No. ONE, and so continue these two (No. TWENTY-SEVEN and No. THIRTY) in alternation, at increasing intervals as the disease improves, until convalescence is established. The diet should be the same as in fevers or inflammation ; only light soups, gruels, toast, etc., in general, and wine, malt-liquor or other stimulants should be strictly avoided.

## CHRONIC DISEASE OF THE KIDNEYS.

Chronic disease of the kidneys may be supposed to exist when we find the following symptoms more or less clearly expressed: The disease may run along for some months, or even years, without being very decided in its symptoms, until the condition of the urine, or the failing health and emaciation of the patient attract attention. The pain in the loins may be only slight, but is increased by pressure on one or both sides in the kidney region. Sometimes the pain extends forward and along down towards the bladder. The urine is discharged frequently, but in diminished quantity. The most important symptom is the condition of the urine; it is thickened, more or less opaque, or loaded with mucus, and often deposits, on standing, a thick, heavy, whitish sediment, in some extreme cases loaded with pus.

TREATMENT.—The Specific No. TWENTY-SEVEN, taken

four times per day, before each meal and on going to rest, two pills at a time, is the proper remedy, and may be continued any length of time with advantage. Sometimes the Specific No. THIRTY may be taken as an intercurrent remedy with benefit.

## INFLAMMATION OF THE BLADDER.—CYSTITIS.

This disease is not very common in its more severe forms, but in its slighter manifestations, is not unfrequently met with. It may be occasioned by the abuse of *cantharides* or other deleterious drugs, or from suppressed piles or the menstrual flow. Also, blows or injuries, or the immoderate use of alcoholic stimulants may excite its appearance. It is known by pain in the bladder, or in the region of that viscus, also by tension, heat and swelling externally; severe pains when the region of the bladder is pressed upon or even touched; frequent and painful discharge of urine, or suppressed, scanty discharge, or frequent, painful or even ineffectual efforts to pass the urine; fever and vomiting are common. When the neck of the bladder is principally involved, the spasms may be so great that the urine is only passed in drops under the most powerful straining, and the bladder becomes distended and mounts like a hard painful ball over the pubic bone in front; if the lower or posterior portion is principally involved, the pain is increased by pressure on the perinæum. The urine is hot, reddish or high colored, but in some cases quite pale. It is rare among young people, and mostly a disease of advanced life.

TREATMENT.—When there is fever, the Specific No. ONE may be given in alternation with No. THIRTY, but in general the latter Specific will be found sufficient alone. Dissolve twelve pellets of No. THIRTY in six large spoonfuls of water, and of these give one every half hour if the pain straining, and distress is very great. But if there is considerable fever, prepare the Specific No. ONE in the same manner, and give the two in alternation at intervals of half an hour at first, and gradually increase the intervals to an hour or two hours, as the disease yields. Hot fomentations to the parts may be of service, should the painful urging and tenesmus be severe.

## CHRONIC INFLAMMATION OF THE BLADDER.

This is usually a disease found among men of somewhat advanced age. There is some diversity in its symptomatic details, but the symptoms are generally as follows: There is an exceedingly irritable condition of the bladder; the patient has frequent calls to urinate, sometimes every half hour or hour. In many cases, and from some slight occasions, a spasm of the neck of the bladder comes on, and notwithstanding the most violent urging, the urine is passed with difficulty or even not at all. In some cases the walls of the bladder become thickened, and hence its capacity very seriously diminished, rendering frequent micturition imperative, and the enlarged and thickened organ may be felt rising like a ball over the pubic bone, and the patient complains of a dull pressure or aching in that region. The urine has frequently an acrid, ammoniacal smell, and is often loaded with mucus.

TREATMENT.—To allay the chronic irritability of the bladder, and restore, if possible, the organ to its natural condition, the Specifics No. TWENTY-SEVEN and No. THIRTY are the proper remedies, and of these two pellets should be taken, in alternation, morning and at night, or even four times per day, taking of No. THIRTY two pellets each morning before breakfast, and afternoon before supper, and of No. TWENTY-SEVEN, each noon before dinner, and at night going to rest.

For an attack of painful or difficult urination, the Specific No. THIRTY should be given in fluid, twelve pellets in six spoonfuls of water, and of these let one spoonful be given every half hour or hour until the pain and spasm has abated and the urine passes freely. Then return again to the Nos. TWENTY-SEVEN and THIRTY for the treatment of the chronic disorder. The Specific No. TEN may often in such cases prove exceedingly beneficial, either alone or in alternation with No. THIRTY.

## GRAVEL—RENAL CALCULI—STONE.

In certain morbid conditions of the kidneys, their functions may be so changed or imperfectly performed, that certain substances which in the healthy condition are discharged in solution, become precipitated, and form hardened concretions, otherwise termed gravel or stone. The deposit is usually first formed in the kidneys, whence sooner or later it makes its way along the ureter into the bladder. These calculi or gravel are of various sizes, forms or material, varying from a pin's head to the size of a pea, or even an egg; some are smooth and roundish, others rough, ragged, irregular, or like scales; more commonly they are reddish chocolate color, or reddish brown, and again are amber color, or again white like chalk; some are easily crushed by the fingers, while others resist the stroke of a hammer. In some cases a calculus becomes deposited in the bladder, and by successive deposits and concretions increases in size until it becomes as large as a walnut or hen's egg, and must be removed by an operation.

These formations may occur in the kidneys, bladder, or even other portions of the urinary passages, but they doubtless originate in the kidneys, and are most frequently found in that organ.

When a gravel passes along the ureter from the kidney

to the bladder, it often gives rise to the most exquisite torture. The patient has the most severe pain in one kidney region, and from thence extending forward and downward along the course of the ureter. The pain comes on in paroxysms with frequent pauses; sometimes the pain extends out over the abdomen, and is attended with fever, nausea, vomiting, and frequent calls to urinate. As soon as the gravel has passed into the bladder the pain ceases. The passage of the gravel from the bladder out is usually far less painful than the passage from the kidney into the bladder.

When a stone occurs in the bladder too large to be passed along the urethra, it is generally manifested by frequent desire to urinate, and pain at the last ejaculations of the urine; the pain is frequently felt at the end of the penis, and there is frequent itching or irritation along the body of this organ; sudden stoppage or arrest of the stream of urine by the stone blocking up the passage, and which may be removed by lying down or a change of position. If the stone is rough and irritating, the urine is frequently mixed with blood, and after a time, piles and prolapsus of the rectum may be occasioned, from the frequent urging and straining to evacuate the bladder.

The causes of the formation of calculus are somewhat obscure, but the disease is most frequently met with among dyspeptics and those living in damp, humid situations, and in cold, variable climates. It is quite common in some families, in others equally rare.

TREATMENT.—*For an attack of gravel* or renal calculi, attended with pain as before mentioned, frequent desire to urinate, etc., give the Specific No. THIRTY, twelve globules in six spoonfuls of water, of which give a spoonful every half hour. Give the patient a hot foot or sitz bath, or apply hot fomentations over the side of the abdomen where the pain is, or give large injections of warm water so as to relax the system and arrest the spasm, and so facilitate the passage of the gravel.

*To prevent the formation* of the calculi, take of the Specific No. THIRTY two pellets at night, and of the No. TWENTY-SEVEN two pellets each morning, and so continue for some months.

Persons afflicted with this disease should subsist as far as possible upon farinaceous food and mucilaginous drinks, in preference to the more heavy and heating meats.

## DIFFICULT, PAINFUL, OR SUPPRESSED URINATION.

We prefer to group together these various conditions of morbid urination, as they frequently arise from the same causes, run into each other in the progress of the complaint, and generally require the same remedies.

*When the urine is retained,* while the kidneys continue to secrete the fluid, the bladder becomes after a few hours so filled and distended, that it rises like a large ball or swelling, immediately over the pubes, which may be perceptible to the touch. The lower portion of the abdomen also becomes swelled and sensitive to pressure. There is some fever, and the inclination to pass water is frequent and urgent, though ineffectual. Should this condition continue any great length of time, inflammation and subsequent mortification may ensue, or the bladder become ruptured with fatal result.

Retention may be caused by inflammation of the urethra, or from stricture, or it may result from suppressed piles. Going too long without urinating, and hence over distention of the bladder may in some cases close the internal orifice of the organ; or it may be occasioned by spasm of the neck of the bladder. Paralysis or inflammation of the neck of the bladder may also produce it. Also tumors in the neck of the bladder, calculus or swelling of the prostate gland.

*Difficulty of discharging the urine* is manifested by frequent desire to urinate, attended with heat, smarting pain, uneasiness and a sense of distention and fullness in the region of the bladder. The urine is only voided in drops or small quantities, sometimes mixed with blood, after great urging or straining.

This condition may be occasioned by gonorrhœa or inflammation of the urethra, spasm of the neck of the bladder, excesses in drinking, exposure to cold in sensitive subjects, suppression of some habitual discharge, presence of gravel in the neck of the bladder or urethra, or from the application of cantharides in the form of a blister. In some rare cases the secretion of urine may be *suppressed*, the kidneys failing to elaborate this secretion from the blood. It mostly occurs in persons of advanced age, or in very young children. It may occur in the course of fevers or in dropsy, or inflammation of some organ of the body. Gouty subjects, particularly after being exposed to cold or wet, or on the suppression of some accustomed discharge, such as hemorrhoids, are most liable to it. Generally there is no inclination to make water, there being no accumulation, and there is no swelling or enlargement in the region of the bladder, indicating an accumulation. Other symptoms are: Nausea, sense of weakness and sinking at the præcordia, sometimes there is also frequent turns of vomiting, severe hiccough, pain in the back, intense headache and restlessness. The skin generally presents a normal condition, but profuse perspiration sometimes supervenes, in some cases with a decided urinous odor. If the secretion is not again established, the system soon suffers, the blood is not deficated, and cerebral symptoms declare themselves, and life terminates in coma.

TREATMENT.—When there is retention of urine, frequent

effort and but little or no discharge, the Specific No. THIRTY should be given dissolved in water, two pellets in a spoonful, and repeated every hour, or even every half hour in urgent cases. Hot fomentations applied to the region of the bladder, and warm seat-baths, are also very efficient auxiliaries.

*Painful, difficult urination* requires nearly the same treatment, only there is no necessity for seat-baths or warm fomentations. The Specific No. THIRTY may be taken, two pills dry on the tongue and repeated every two or three hours, will be sufficient in most cases. Should there be calculus, tumors, or other mechanical obstructions in the neck of the bladder or urethra, the case will be more obstinate, yet the use of the medicine and warm fomentations will be proper, and generally efficient. If there is inflammation of the urethra, the same treatment as in gonorrhœa must be pursued.

When the secretion of the kidneys appears *scanty* or *suppressed*, a few portions of the Specific No. ELEVEN, either alone or in alternation with No. THIRTY, at intervals of two or three hours, will be probably sufficient to restore the secretion again.

## URINARY INCONTINENCE—WETTING THE BED.

This difficulty is manifested in a frequent desire to pass off the water, and an inability to retain it for any length of time after the inclination comes on. Sometimes the call comes on every hour, or even more frequently during the day, and the urgency is very pressing. It may arise from weakness or relaxation of the neck of the bladder, or from the urine being too acrid or irritating, or from the presence of gravel, or some diseased condition of the bladder itself.

A frequent phase of this disease manifests itself in the

involuntary discharge of the urine at night, or what is termed "wetting the bed." It it mostly noticed amorg children under ten or twelve years of age, but has occasionally been known to continue to adult age. Sometimes it appears in children apparently disconnected from any other morbid condition of the urinary organs; the child has perfect control while awake, but during the unconsciousness of sleep the system becomes relaxed and the urine is passed involuntarily. It may arise in some cases from the irritation of worms, or from the secretion being too acrid, but in general its foundation, especially in obstinate cases, will be found in a scrofulous diathesis.

TREATMENT.—In all cases of frequent calls to urinate or inability to retain the secretion, the Specific No. THIRTY, two pellets three times per day, will be sufficient, and be found promptly curative.

When the disease may be supposed to arise from the irritation of worms, the Specific No. Two may be given in alternation with No. THIRTY each taken twice in the course of the day.

In obstinate cases of wetting the bed, the Specific No. TWENTY-TWO should be given, two pellets every morning on rising, and the No. THIRTY, two pellets at night, and this course pursued until the cure is effected.

In the case of children subject to this infirmity, care should be taken not to let them drink of water or other fluid late in the evening, or on going to bed; not to permit them to eat apples, acid fruits, watermelons or cantelopes late in the afternoon or evening, and to use no kind of drink calculated to stimulate the urinary secretion; and also when children are subject to this infirmity, to have them urinate the last thing before retiring, and also very early in the morning, and on no account suffer them to lie in the wet clothes.

## EXCESSIVE SECRETION OF URINE—DIABETES.

This disease consists of an immoderate secretion of urine, which, when fully developed, contains a large proportion of saccharine matter. Sometimes, in the earlier stages of the disease, and even in some forms of it, the saccharine principle is wanting, and the urine presents mainly the characteristic of excessive quantity, and being of generally pale or straw colored. When there is evidently sugar in the urine, which may be known by its greater specific gravity, or by evaporating it, and it is always a dangerons, and very generally ultimately a fatal disease. The disease comes on slowly, more commonly in men than in women, and is manifested by an immoderate discharge of pale, watery, straw-colored urine, sometimes amounting to several quarts in the twenty-four hours; intense thirst and voracious appetite, which are found difficult to satisfy, although there is very generally some derangement of the digestion. There is sometimes pain or distress in the lumbar region, or a sense of distressing weakness in that region. If the disease progresses, and especially in the form called *diabetes melletis* or sugary urine, the body becomes pale and emaciated, thirst excessive, the quantity of urine discharged exceeds the amount of fluid and aliment taken into the system; the sense of prostration increases, the pulse becomes rapid and weak; the breathing laborious, and dropsical effusion of the lower extremities occur.

The disease may run from a few weeks to two or more years, makes frequent pauses and then resumes its course, but sooner or later claims its victim. It is generally found among persons with shattered constitutions, who have injured themselves by excesses, or by drains upon the system, or intemperance in eating or drinking, or those who have suffered depletion from the abuse of cathartics or bleedings.

TREATMENT.—The diet is of the utmost consequence. Everything must be prohibited which contains the saccharine principle. Potatoes, fruits, milk, as well as substances that excite the action of the kidneys, must be prohibited. Animal food must form the staple of diet. Beef, mutton, venison, are best. Let the little bread eaten be well toasted and stale, and as little of any kind of vegetables as possible. As to medical treatment, I have found *Phus. acid, Carbo veg.*, and *Nat. mur.* the best remedies, and give them in a low form, first or third attenuation five drops three times per day.

## HEMORRHAGE WITH THE URINE—HEMATURIA.

Occasionally the urine is found of a more or less deeply reddish tinge, and an examination shows the presence of blood. Sometimes quite a proportion of the discharge consists of blood, and at other times there is but a slight admixture. It may arise from any cause that separates any of the minute blood vessels along its course. Thus, falls, blows, bruises, leaping, running, any violent exercise, or the lodgment of a stone in the kidney, urethra, or bladder, or an inflammation of the kidney may occasion it. Irregular menstruation, suppression of piles, excessive indulgence in spirituous drinks, venereal excesses, the use of asparagus or cantharides may at times induce it.

When the blood is discharged in streaks or dots, and deposits, on standing a dark brown sediment like coffee grounds, it is likely to have come from the irritating effects of a stone in the bladder, and the act of urinating is attended with some straining and effort. If it proceeds from the kidneys, there will be pain in the lumbar region, anxiety, numbness along the inside of one or both thighs; drawing up of the testicles, and derangement of the bowels.

The presence of blood in the urine is always a serious matter, and should demand our attention. In most cases it is controllable, but should not be neglected.

TREATMENT.—The Specific No. THIRTY will generally be found sufficient, and should always be tried first, two pellets dissolved in a spoonful of water, and given every two or three hours, gradually increasing the intervals as the disease yields.

Should the disease arise from the kidneys, and especially if there should be an appearance of pus or matter in the secretion, it will be better to alternate the Specifics No. TWENTY-SEVEN and No. THIRTY, two pellets at a time, and say four times per day, and let this course be continued for some weeks.

Drinking of cold water during this complaint is objectionable, and tends to increase the irritation already existing. Barley-water in large quantities is the best drink.

Should these remedies not control the disease, and especially if the amount of blood in the urine is quite copious, half a teaspoonful of WITCH HAZEL, taken every one or two hours, will be effectual.

# DISEASES OF WOMEN.

## MENSTRUATION.

The sufferings attendant upon the various forms of disease to which women are particularly liable, comprise a large share of the evils to which they are subject. Much of the health and happiness of the sex depends upon the proper performance of the various functions incident to their peculiar systems. No considerable derangement in these functions can exist for any length of time, without drawing the entire system into sympathetic suffering. While this class of diseases is so important, and exercise so grave an influence over the health and happiness of the female, yet their nature is such as to necessarily exclude them, to a great extent, from observation, and the victim often prefers to suffer the pain, distress and inconvenience of them, than to disclose them to her medical attendant. It is then especially important that ladies, and especially mothers, should make themselves acquainted with the subject, and as far as possible to be able to correct these disturbances in their earlier stages, and before they have become complicated or inveterate from lapse of time.

The first menses usually make their appearance in this climate at about the fifteenth year; in warm climates earlier, and in colder later. It is also subject to variations, depending upon the general health, vigor, and development of the person. For a year or two it may be scanty, and not unfrequently subject to some irregularities, which need not excite apprehension, unless they are very grave or important. In healthy women it should appear every twenty-eight days, and flow four or five days, varying again according to the health and vigor of the person. About the forty-fifth year of life it generally ceases altogether, though in some cases it may commence with irregularities some years earlier, and in others the function may continue regularly until the fiftieth year, or even later. Its cessation is marked by irregularities and various disturbances of the system, extending for months, or even years. This cessation of the monthly flows, and the disturbances of the period, are generally termed the "change of life" or the critical period.

## TARDY MENSES—DELAYING MENSES.

When menstruation in young girls does not come on at the usual time, it is not always proper to hasten to administer medicine, with a view of forcing their appearance. It is a better rule, so long as the general health remains good, to do nothing to promote this secretion, beyond attention to the proper clothing, exercise, and diet of the patient. The clothing should be warm and changed to suit the temperature and season, and a wholesome, generous diet should be adopted, avoiding all spices, coffee, and high-seasoned food. Care should be likewise exercised that the child be not overtaxed by study, too long or too severe lessons, or sitting too long at the piano, while, from want of appetite, or unsuitable or too meagre diet, the system is insufficiently nourished during this period. These measures will generally be sufficient. Should they however fail, or should there be some symptoms of its approach, such as flushes of heat, frequent giddiness of the head, heaviness in the abdomen and about the loins, or if she is dull, stupid, melancholy or sad; or if she is bloated, sluggish, or even if very slender and feeble, the case should demand attention, and the patient should receive proper care in order to prevent after diseases, irregularity and suffering.

Treatment.—The Specific No. Eleven, two pellets night and morning, will be found sufficient, and may be continued regularly until the menses are established. Fresh air, moderate exercise, and simple, generous diet, are important. A sponge bath night and morning, avoiding exposure to night air and cold damp feet, are also important auxiliaries.

## CHLOROSIS—GREEN SICKNESS.

In some cases the menses fail to appear at the proper age, or appear imperfectly, very scanty in quantity, wanting in proper color, and irregularly as to time, or not at all, and in addition there is more or less of the following symptoms: Weariness, want of strength or vigor, languor, debility, the patient becomes emaciated, face pale, earthy, lips blanched, bloodless, or sometimes flushes of heat, depraved appetite, longing for sharp, acid, or cheering things, or for slate, chalk, or clay. The bowels are irregular, confined, or relaxed; abdomen often distended, with borborigmi or flatulence, especially after eating, or along in the latter part of the day; limbs frequently are swelled and cold; headache, short breath, and palpitation of the heart on slight exercise, and not unfrequently, short, dry cough. These symptoms in young girls are always of the utmost importance, and demand care and attention for their removal. Yet you should not rush to extreme means. A little time, patience and care, with the use of the proper medicines, will generally bring all around right, and give the patient a good, healthy constitution.

Treatment.—The Specific No. Eleven, two pellets in water, three times per day, will almost always be found sufficient, and especially if coupled with this, due care be exercised with regard to the diet and regimen of the patient. All that has been said under the previous section in regard to *Tardy Menstruation* obtains here. Good air, generous diet, warm clothing, daily frictions of the body and bathing, are all means to establish and build up the general health, and most important and efficient auxiliaries in the work of restoration, and generally succeed in a few months in restoring the patient, and bringing her over this oftentimes critical period. Other medicines may be used as intercurrent remedies in the treatment, if the symptoms so require: as, the No. TEN for flatulence, feeble digestion and poor appetite, No. SEVEN for cough or hoarseness, No. ONE or No. THIRTY-FIVE for flushes of heat or headache. These remedies may be given, one or two doses of two pellets per day, while the No. ELEVEN is given regularly night or morning

## SCANTY, INSUFFICIENT MENSES.

In some cases after menstruation is established, the discharge does not appear at the proper time, there being five or six or more weeks between the intervals; or it may continue only for a day or two, being pale or unusual in color, or stopping, and then coming on again for a few hours; or other features of irregularity, denoting an unhealthy or feeble menstrual flow. All such cases indicate either general debility, feebleness of the entire system, the presence of some serious disease or derangement of the uterine system, and demand attention. We should seek to build up the general health, by nourishing food, stimulants in rare cases, good air and healthful exercise, keeping the feet dry and warm, and the lower extremities well protected, and the mind cheerful and happy.

Beside these hygienic observances, the use of the Specific No. ELEVEN, two pellets night and morning, or even two pellets before each meal and on going to rest at night, will in general restore the system to its natural and healthy function.

## SUPPRESSED MENSES.

Sometimes, in regularly menstruating women, the discharge becomes suppressed, and fails to appear at the proper time. This is most commonly the result of cold, and especially of *damp cold,* and is a cause to which women should be constantly on their guard. Cold feet, getting the feet wet, insufficient covering for the feet, legs and lower abdomen, or a thorough chilling of the whole body about the time it should appear, or even during the flow, are sufficient to arrest the discharge, and result in very mischievous consequences. Sudden and powerful emotions of the mind, or grief and desponding, may also arrest it, and at times, these powerful influences applied during the intervals between the periods, may be sufficient to prevent its appearance. The use of acids, vinegar, pickles, or harsh, indigestible things, may have a similar effect. When these obstructing causes are applied during the flow, or just at the time of its being established, the consequences are much more severe and violent than when they are applied during the interval.

But when the obstructing causes are applied during the interval, a train of symptoms arise which are quite as serious, if not as sudden and violent. The patient becomes pale, languid, debilitated; her appetite fails, and she looks sickly and dejected; there is loss of energy and ambition; the feet and ankles often swell; she becomes nervous, palpitation of the heart, indigestion, flatulence, and shortness of breath appear, and very generally leucorrhœa comes on. In feeble persons predisposed to consumption or pulmonary disease, suppression is peculiarly prejudicial, and always demand serious attention. The result is that: The flow may either cease suddenly, or it may not come on at all at the next period, or it may come on attended with scanty, irregular discharge, or with severe pain and distress. In the worst cases we have frightful attacks of spasmodic pains in the bowels and stomach, often attended with retching, vomiting, headache, flushed face, delirium, convulsions, hysteria, palpitation of the heart, or difficult breathing, etc.

TREATMENT.—Dissolve at once twelve pills of Specific No. ELEVEN, in six dessert spoonfuls of water, and of this give one spoonful every hour, giving the patient also a hot foot-bath, and putting her quietly and comfortably to bed if the case is sufficiently serious to justify it. This will generally suffice; if it does not, another dose may be prepared in the same manner, and taken at intervals of two or three hours, until the result is accomplished.

If the flow has been fully established, it may not be requisite to do anything in the interval. But if the result has been imperfectly accomplished, the Specific No. ELEVEN should be given, two pellets every two or three nights during the interval, and at the time it should again appear, care should be taken that there be no exposure or danger of a chill to prevent its appearance.

WHEN THE PROPER TIME RETURNS, and the menses do not appear, take two of the pills for IRREGULARITIES every night on going to bed, and bathe the feet in warm water fifteen or twenty minutes, for two or three nights in succession, if necessary. A single dose or two will, however, usually be found successful.

## PAINFUL MENSTRUATION.

Many women suffer an untold amount of *pain* at every return of the menstrual period, not only bearing down, but cuttings, gripings, colic, cramps, and, in some cases, even convulsions attend every access of menstruation. Often these sufferings are so excruciating as to embitter the life of the patient, and cause her to dread even the thought of a menstrual return; and the prostrating effects of one period are hardly recovered from, before another comes on. These sufferings are liable to occur during every period of life, from the commencement to the close of menstruation, and certain persons or constitutions are peculiarly predisposed to them. Exposure to cold and want of proper care during the first years of menstruation, are the common sources of this suffering. The pain often begins some hours, or even days before the flow commences, and at other times the discharge commences and continues several hours, then diminishes or ceases entirely, with great suffering. The pains may continue an indefinite period, ceasing or becoming less when the flow has been established under proper treatment, or they may continue during the entire period, without shortening the period, or diminishing the quantity. The pains may be of an intermitting, expulsive character, or a steady, aching pain in the loins, hips, and back, like those which usually precede menstruation. In some cases membranous shreds are expelled, and in others the flow is natural. Not unfrequently the breasts are swelled, sensitive, or even quite painful.

Such cases are sometimes found in connection with scanty, retarded, or irregular periods; and again, with regular or too abundant discharge, the feature being excessively violent pain, pressure, bearing down, and even cramps and convulsions at every access of the monthly period. Pen cannot express the anguish and pain suffered by some women at every menstrual return.

TREATMENT.—*During the interval* between the periods, give every night two pellets of the Specific No. ELEVEN.

*When the pain comes on,* give two pellets of the Specific No. THIRTY-ONE, every one or two hours, until relief is obtained, or several hours have passed. If not fully relieved by this, give the Specific No. ELEVEN, in alternation with No. THIRTY-ONE, and at the same intervals. In some cases where there is great bearing down, or when the discharge is quite profuse, the Specific No. THIRTY-FIVE will be found very efficient, given in the same manner, either alone or in alternation with No. THIRTY-ONE. This course will very generally relieve the most inveterate cases.

*For headache during the menses,* take the Specific No. ELEVEN, every two hours two pellets, until relieved. In some cases the Specific No. THIRTY-TWO, taken in the same manner, acts like a charm.

## TOO PROFUSE, OR TOO FREQUENT MENSES.

Often, especially in women subject to the whites, and dependent also upon a similar relaxed condition in the system, the menses are *too profuse,* returning again after a cessation of only ten, fourteen, or sixteen days, and flowing from five to ten days. Thus the discharge may not only be *too* profuse, but also *too* soon and too frequent, or it may only appear too soon, without being for the time excessive in quantity. Sometimes the secretion is scanty for some days, and then comes on like a flood, causing great prostration, faintness and debility, from which the patient has scarcely time to recover, before a new attack comes on. It may be attended with only slight pain or distress beyond the sensation of debility, consequent upon the great drain upon the system. But in other cases the pain, distress, or dragging down pains are very severe and exhausting. Sometimes, indeed, the discharge is so profuse as to merit the designation of real hemorrhage, or flooding, and, of course, induces a condition of great debility and prostration. Women subject to this difficulty, should entirely abstain from coffee, wine, or other stimulants, and also from all heating drinks, spices, or condiments so long as there is danger from this source. These excitements exert a direct influence in keeping up the irritation of the uterus, and in promoting this unhealthy flow.

TREATMENT.—During the interval between the periods, the Specific No. TWELVE, two pellets morning and night, should be taken, regulating the diet as above directed. After the flow has continued two or three days, and if desirable to arrest its further excess, then commence the use of the Specifics No. TEN and No. TWELVE in alternation, giving two pellets at a time at intervals of six hours. If the discharge is very profuse from the first, the two above Specifics may be commenced earlier, and may be given every four hours in alternation. When the discharge lingers along for several days, two or three pellets of No. TEN, given at night, will generally suffice to arrest it.

In case there be at any time an excessive flow, amounting to a dangerous hemorrhage, from whatever cause, ten or twelve pellets of Specific No. TWELVE should be dissolved in six spoonfuls of water, and one spoonful should be taken every hour, until the dangerous symptoms are warded off, when the medicine may be administered at longer intervals. It will be obvious that the patient must remain perfectly quiet, and abstain from warm drinks, or any excitement at such times.

## CESSATION OF THE MENSES.

This period, which is very frequently termed the CHANGE OF LIFE, occurs most commonly at or about the forty-fifth year. In some cases where menstruation has commenced early, and the person has lived luxuriously, it may terminate as early as thirty-seven, forty, or the forty-second year, and in other cases, with strong, vigorous ladies, the menses often continue to the forty-eighth or fiftieth year, or even a more advanced period of life.

Its approach is usually manifested by some irregularities in the monthly flow. It may come on too soon, or be delayed one, two, or more weeks, and the discharge may manifest some change, being in some cases light or pale, being largely mixed with mucus, and in others being very profuse, not unfrequently amounting to profuse and alarming hemorrhages. Sometimes the flow comes on suddenly, and again ceases without warning, and unattended by bad symptoms. In some cases the change comes on so gradual and free from constitutional disturbance, that before the subject is fully aware of it, she has ceased to menstruate, and has safely glided over this troublesome passage into the serene ocean of after life, exempt from many sufferings and frailties to which she had previously been exposed.

More frequently, however, as women approach this period, they have turns of vertigo, headache, flushes of heat, occasional palpitation of the heart, more or less nervousness and some sense of debility; sometimes frequent passage of pale urine in large quantities, or of high-colored, scanty urine; pain in the lower part of the abdomen, back and hips, or extending down the thighs; heat in the lower part of the stomach and back; piles may be troublesome and bleed freely; swelling of the lower limbs or abdomen, which subside without the usual symptoms of flatulence, and pruritis or violent itching of the organs is not uncommon. This range of symptoms may appear in whole or only in part, or be variously modified in particular cases.

Treatment.—So long as the health is good, and the monthly flow is gradually diminishing from month to month, medicine is not required, but in all cases a proper diet and regimen is important. The diet should be simple, avoiding all stimulants, and all highly-seasoned stimulating meats, and using chiefly vegetable and farinaceous articles of food; frequent exercise in the open air in suitable weather, bathing, and the proper culture of the skin should not be neglected. The dress should be so regulated as to suitably protect the person, and prevent unnecessary exposure to the necessities of climate; and sleeping, also, in heated rooms, and on soft, heating beds, should be avoided. The Specific No. THIRTY-TWO, two pellets morning and night, will be generally efficient in arresting nearly all the disturbances arising during this period. Should there occur at any time such a discharge as to be serious or threaten a hemorrhage, rest, quiet, and the use of the Specific No. TWELVE, in alternation with No. THIRTY-TWO, two pellets every hour, will promptly avert any danger. No fear need be entertained from the long-continued use of the Specific No. THIRTY-TWO during this period, as it may be used for months or years without prejudice.

## LEUCORRHŒA OR WHITES.

Few affections of women are more common than this, and, perhaps, none more annoying. It consists of a discharge from the genital organs, mostly whitish, but not unfrequently discolored, and of varying nature and consistency. It most frequently occurs between the ages of puberty and the cessation of the menses, yet it is not uncommon in little girls or even young children, and occasionally met with in quite old women. Some persons and families are much more subject to it than others; those subject to catarrhs, and of relaxed habit of body, being most liable. The more common exciting causes are difficult or tedious labors, the immoderate use of the organs, late hours, abuse of tea, coffee and spices, luxurious living, and sometimes the neglect of proper bathings. When it appears in children, the cause is generally seat-worms, neglect of proper bathings, or some irritating matter or substance applied to the parts. This discharge is also most profuse just before and after the menstrual period, and during pregnancy. It may be trifling ,or quite profuse, and its character may vary as much as its quantity. At the commencement it may be only a slight increase of the natural, healthy, transparent mucus, but it gradually becomes more dense, thick and gelatinous, or it may become thin, milky, or acrid, at times rendering the parts sore or excoriated; in many cases it is yellowish and purulent; or again it may be greenish or even a brownish hue. The discharge often is not constant, but irregular, or by emissions. At first, and while the discharge is trifling, the system seems to feel the loss but slightly, but after a time the results begin to manifest themselves by constant pain in the back and loins; aching in the hips; bearing down or sense of weight low in the abdomen; pale face; coldness of the extremities; despondency or low spirits; loss of appetite; rising of wind or food; nervous symptoms, neuralgy, and similar consensual manifestations. Leucorrhœa should always demand attention. On the first intimation of its approach, the subject should at once avoid the exciting causes, and apply the proper Specifics, and thus arrest in the commencement what might otherwise become an intolerable burden, or the forerunner of some serious uterine affection. Not unfrequently it is the symptom of some disease of the uterus which demands prompt and efficient aid, and the commencement is the best time to arrest it.

TREATMENT.—Persons subject to this disease should carefully protect the feet and lower abdomen from sudden changes of temperature and colds, by wearing firm, substantial covering for the feet, and underclothing, avoid standing on the cold, wet ground, take moderate exercise in the open air, avoid over-heated rooms, coffee, exciting drinks or highly-spiced food, and should take of the Specific No. TWELVE, two pellets night and morning. If the bowels are also inclined to constipation, the Specific No. TEN, two pills may be taken at night, and the No. TWELVE morning and at noon.

When leucorrhœa exists in connection with too scanty, infrequent or irregular menses, the Specific No. ELEVEN deserves a preference, and may be taken two pellets three times per day.

When it exists in little girls or young children, a careful examination should be made for the small pin worms which may sometimes be found lodged within the parts, and which should be removed by frequent bathings, and the child treated for worms, by giving the Specific No. Two each morning and the Specific No. TWELVE at night, two pellets at a time.

## PROLAPSUS UTERI—FALLING OF THE WOMB.

This is also a very common complaint among women, affecting in a greater or lesser extent quite a proportion of the sex. Sometimes it is only a passing and comparatively trivial affection, coming on from some severe fatigue or over exertion, and soon passing off from rest and a recumbent posture, while at others it is a constant and chronic affection, forbidding any considerable effort, and sometimes confining the patient to her room. The immediate causes of the prolapsus are various, among which the principal are: Getting up too soon after confinement; results of over-lifting or over-straining, or of falls; very severe coughs or vomitings; tight lacing, and a more or less relaxed habit of body, and added to this, a more or less engorged or congested condition of the uterus itself. It is usually attended with a feeling of weight and heaviness low down in the abdomen; lameness or pain in the back and loins, dragging in the groins; a benumbing sensation extending down the limbs; a sensation as if everything would be pressed out while standing on the feet; a sensation also of emptiness, faintness, or "goneness" at the pit of the stomach; and often some difficulty in passing water or when at stool. In some severe cases there is difficulty in rising to the feet, and the patient must lean forward and support herself by placing her hands upon her thighs. All these sufferings are aggravated by standing or walking, and disappear or are relieved by lying down. There is also in many cases, a constant discharge of mucus from the parts, often unhealthy and abundant, and the monthly period is generally too profuse, all of which contribute to increase the nervous debility, and exhaust the strength of the patient.

TREATMENT.—In many instances, and in all the less aggravated cases, the use of medicines in the form of proper Specifics will be sufficient to remove the difficulty, if the patient will follow the treatment persistently, and avoid the exciting causes of the disease. But there may be cases so situated that mechanical aid in the form of some of the various "pessaries" or "supporters" is indispensable. But I think we should never resort to these until we have exhausted other means, as once introduced, they may and most likely will become a life-long companion. When the symptoms are present, indicating a prolapsed condition, or those above described, the Specifics No. THIRTY-FIVE and No. TEN are the most efficient remedies and should be administered, two pellets of No. THIRTY-FIVE each morning, and the same of No. TEN at night in all the milder cases. When the symptoms are more severe and decided, the pellets may be dissolved in water and administered as often as once in four hours, being at the same time careful to give the patient all the rest and quiet possible. When the displacement is severe and decided, and especially when it is the result of a recent strain, overlifting or accident, the patient should lie down upon the back with the limbs drawn up and endeavor to replace the organ, and then maintain the position until the organ has, in a degree, resumed its position, and the pains and dragging sensation has disappeared.

When prolapsus occurs in connection with chronic leucorrhœa, the Specifics No. TEN and No. TWELVE should be administered, giving each morning and afternoon, two pellets of No. TWELVE, and at each noon and at night the same of No. TEN until this condition is radically removed.

## HYSTERIA.

Ladies between the ages of fifteen and thirty and more especially the unmarried, are subject to attacks of hysteria, which are in general connected with some anomalies in the menstruation, and mostly occur in connection with that period. The form and succession of symptoms are almost innumerable, since there is scarcely a form of disease that hysteria has not been known to similate. The more frequent symptoms, however, are those of anxiety, depression, weeping; difficult or oppressed breathing; palpitation or nausea; sensation as if there was a ball in the throat, which proceeds from a pain in the left side; sometimes there is twisting or turning of the body, rigid, stiff limbs and clenching of the teeth. Then there are fits of laughing, crying, screaming, incoherent talking or frothing at the mouth, or hiccough. Sometimes an attack commences with violent spasmodic pain in the back, which may extend to the chest or stomach, with cold perspiration, pale, earthy face and weak, thread-like pulse. An attack lasts from a few minutes to several hours, and passes off with eructations, sighing, sobbing, and a sense of soreness in the whole body. It is quite common in some families and individuals, and it may be excited by sudden emotions. The predisposition to it is increased by an inactive life, free use of stimulants, or depressing mental condition.

TREATMENT.—The predisposition should be overcome by correcting any unhealthy or unusual condition of the menstrual function, and by an active, cheerful life. For an attack of hysteria in the more common form, the Specific No. THREE, two pellets every half hour or hour, will generally suffice. If connected with scanty menstruation, administer the Specific No. ELEVEN in the same manner. If there are attacks of cramps similating, or actual convulsions, administer the Specific No. THIRTY-THREE, two pellets every hour until relieved.

## INFLAMMATION OF THE LABIA.

An inflammation of the external organs of women occasionally occurs, during which one of the labia becomes swelled, hard, red and painful and sensitive to motion. In some cases a swelling and suppuration and discharge similar to that of a boil occurs, all of which is very painful and tedious. In some persons there have been frequent repetitions of the same phenomenon. It may be occasioned by the rupture of the hymen, or from injury in the newly married, or come on as a consequence of tedious labors, or in other cases from some morbid condition of the system developing itself in this direction.

TREATMENT.—When it is the result of violence or injury to the parts, the WITCH HAZEL, diluted one-half with water, and applied to the part by a cloth saturated with the lotion, will give very prompt and decided relief, and the

Specific No. ONE, two pills every two or three hours, may also be taken upon the tongue, and continued until the heat, swelling and pain has subsided. In cases where it assumes the nature of a boil, and suppuration occurs or is inevitable, the Specific No. TWENTY-TWO may be given, two pellets every four or six hours, until cured. An occasional dose will prevent a return.

## PREGNANCY.

This period may be considered as perhaps the most important era in the life of woman. She is now no longer acting for herself alone, but becomes invested with a new and serious responsibility, as upon her well or ill doing during this period may depend the future health and happiness of another, to whom she stands at once in the most endearing and most responsible relation. Experience, and the ample records of the most careful observers have clearly shown that the physical, mental, and even moral constitution of the future being is greatly modified, and in some instances formed, by the condition of the mother during this interesting period. Keeping this in view, we shall endeavor to point out for mothers that general course of conduct which will be most likely to secure for themselves ease and safety during the approaching trial, and for the offspring, that physical and mental condition which will best fit them for the duties of life. Should these slight restrictions involve some self-denials or restraints, they will be assured that they will be more than repaid in their own welfare in the near future, and in the consciousness of having so truly contributed to the health and happiness of another.

The most common causes of weak and sickly offsprings are: Ill health or constitutional taint of one or both parents; very early or very late marriages; too great inequality between the ages of the parents; errors in dress, diet, and general habits of life; and finally powerful mental emotions.

Fortunately, under the benign and yet potent influence of our system of treatment, not only long standing diseases, but also hereditary taints may be entirely overcome and eradicated, so that we have less to fear than formerly in regard to their transmission to offspring. And it may as well be remarked here, that the intermarriage of relations or members of the same family, always aggravates and perpetuates any particular fault or vice of either parent, even though in some cases it may disappear in one generation, only to reappear in greater violence or strength in a succeeding one, while by judicious intermarriage with persons of opposite temperaments, the fault or vice is constantly found to diminish.

It is not advisable for women in this country to enter the marriage relation before the twenty-first or twenty-second year, though it is undeniable that many have become strong, healthy mothers, lived to old age, and have reared large families of healthy children, who have married at a much earlier age; yet prior to this period, the organism is rarely fully developed and confirmed, and those who marry at sixteen or eighteen years of age, incur some hazard of severe after suffering to themselves, and of giving birth to weak and delicate children. Not unfrequently the children of very early marriages perish in infancy, or after contending with the various diseases of infancy in continual delicacy, sink into a premature grave. Women who marry late in life incur considerable personal risk, and their offspring are rarely healthy. The children of old men, though by a young wife, are often extremely delicate and very susceptible to illness, and not unfrequently precede their father to the grave, or linger but to drag out a miserable and wearisome existence.

Pregnancy should not be considered a state of disease,

but as a natural function, and one in which nature has taken great care to have as perfect in all its appointments, and as free from suffering as possible. While pregnancy runs its equable and uniform course, the expectant mother enjoys an almost complete exemption from prevailing epidemic, or even infectious diseases, and we likewise find that during its course chronic diseases are frequently suspended or modified. With the exception of some slight morning sickness, or other trifling uneasiness, a well constituted organism should enjoy as good health during this period as at any other. Thousands pass through it, giving birth to healthy and vigorous children without even the most trifling inconvenience or suffering. Though nature has taken kind care to render this season as far as possible exempt from disease on the part of the mother, and to provide for the health and welfare of the future being, yet in many instances her kind intentions are frustrated by the direct infraction of her laws. The expectant mother should therefore bear in mind the duty of leading, as far as possible, a regular and systematic course of life, since its violation may fall with fearful severity upon the helpless infant.

Air and Exercise.—Preservation and enjoyment of the highest health are dependent upon nothing more than the two points mentioned above, yet, perhaps, in nothing are there more frequent errors. Neither air nor exercise is individually sufficient. Those who, from habit or fashion, merely take the air in their carriages, and shun the slightest physical exercise, either from habits or from acquired indolence, can scarcely expect to derive the benefit which nature has annexed to the observation of her laws, in a course of pregnancy, free from suffering, and the production of fully developed and healthy offspring.

During this period, therefore, passive or carriage exercise is not sufficient; on the contrary, continual passive exercise in a carriage has been found particularly injurious during and towards the end of the second period of pregnancy, and is frequently the cause of premature or abnormal births. Exercise on horseback, even without taking into consideration the risk of fright or accident to the rider, and the fearful consequences that may therefrom result, is still more objectionable for many reasons. Walking, and that frequently in the open air, only meets every indication, as it not only brings the whole of the organic muscles into play, and imparts tone and strength to them by their exercise, but likewise impart the increased vigor and energy of the mother to her offspring.

Another class, that of thrifty housewives, take a great deal of exercise, but without corresponding benefit, as it is mostly within doors, and in many cases these women, either from activity of temperament or the seeming necessities of their position, frequently over-fatigue themselves, rise early, toil constantly, retire late and frequently slumber unrefreshingly, and in this manner undermine their organic powers, to their own permanent loss and injury, and that of their offspring.

There are still others who not unfrequently injure their health, or bring on a miscarriage through excessive levity and thoughtlessness, by unrestrained indulgence in active exercise, running, romping, riding on horseback, dancing, etc. Such should remember that a miscarriage once or twice induced is likely to return again upon the slightest provocation, and that, when several have taken place, the greatest care and skill are required, even if it be possible to enable her to attain her full time, and that frequent casualties of this nature not unfrequently undermine the constitution, or terminate in that serious and painful disease, uterine cancer.

The best exercise, therefore, for a person during this period, is walking every day when the weather permits, in the open air. In order to prove beneficial and not to interfere with digestion, exercise should be taken two or three hours after a moderate meal, about midday, or in the afternoon, except during hot weather, when the morning or the evening may be preferred, taking care to avoid the night damps by not remaining out too late.

CLOTHING.—The dress of the expectant woman should of course be suited to the season, and in passing from a warm to a cold atmosphere, the throat and neck should be well protected, to avoid the risk of taking cold. But a point of far greater importance is the adaptation of clothing to her form, so as to preclude all unnecessary pressure upon any part of the frame calculated to interfere with the functions of those important organs which are destined for the birth and nourishment of the infant; tight lacing, therefore, at all times most objectionable, is peculiarly so at this period, inasmuch as it cramps the natural action of the body, and bearing directly upon the abdominal muscles, the blood-vessels, the lymphatics, and the whole intestinal economy, produces narrowness of the chest, disturbed circulation, and induration or other derangements of the liver, and exercises a most baneful influence upon the breasts and uterus. We should bear in mind that pressure upon these organs during development takes place in direct contravention of the operations of nature. Ladies in their efforts to preserve the elegance of their shape during pregnancy, are little aware that the constricting force thus exercised upon the abdominal muscles, destroys their elasticity, prevents a proper retraction after parturition, and thus proves one of the most common causes of permanent abdominal deformity. Besides, to the culpable vanity of their mothers in this and other respects, many, it is probable, owe their club-feet and other malformations; and in addition to these evils, this practice not unfrequently deranges the position of the fœtus, a displacement, which, in addition to the consequent want of energy in the muscles of the parts concerned, often results in protracted and dangerous labors. Besides, this tight lacing is liable to produce a premature labor. To tight lacing also may be attributed the difficulty which many women experience in suckling their children, from the incipient process required for the subsequent secretion of milk having been interfered with by the unnatural pressure upon the beautifully constructed mechanism of the breasts. From this, also, sometimes arises cancers and other affections of the breast, and also the retraction and diminution of the nipple from which the act of suckling is rendered difficult, and in some cases impossible. Young girls of seventeen or eighteen are frequently found with pendulous breasts, owing to an artificial support having usurped the office of muscles intended by nature for that purpose, thus throwing them out of employment. Garters too tightly bound are generally injurious, more particularly to pregnant females, as the pressure thus exercised upon the blood vessels tends to the development of varicose veins in the inferior extremities, (to which the system is already sufficiently predisposed,) which thus, in many instances, become painful and troublesome.

DIET.—The greatest simplicity should be observed in regard to food. The quantity should be such as to afford a generous nutrition for the system, while an excess is prejudicial, causing dyspepsia and general uneasiness, and from its mechanical effects acting injuriously upon the fœtus, which also shares in any derangements of the mother.

The *quality* of her food is important; everything possessing a medicinal property should be avoided, and only that selected which is simply nutritive. Coffee and green tea should be wholly abandoned, and black tea in moderation should be used if any. Wines, liquors, beer, or other stimulating beverages are injurious. Where women have been long accustomed to them, a little good wine may perhaps be taken daily, but the better rule is to avoid stimulants of every kind altogether.

Mental Employment and General Habits.—While the body should be maintained in a condition of health, the mind also should be kept in a state of serenity. An easy cheerfulness of temper, and freedom from oppressive care and anxiety, are essential to the well-being of the unborn infant. It is well settled, from repeated observation, that the predominant feeling or tone of mind of the mother has often cast its shade over the future mental organization of the child, and this fact illustrates the importance of keeping the mind properly occupied during this period, and that its meditations should be cheerful and free from depressing influences and gloomy forebodings on the one hand, and the levity, frivolity, and excitements of fashionable dissipation on the other. Nothing can well be more injurious to the future physical and mental well-being of the child, than a round of giddy dissipation, late hours, and fashionable excitement, in connection with physical indolence and inactivity.

Influence of External Objects upon the Unborn Infant.—"The effect of any unpleasant or unsightly object upon the imagination of the mother, and the transmission of that effect to the offspring, as manifested in various mental or physical peculiarities after birth, is a theory as old as tradition. Without entering into the various arguments both for and against it, we simply advise expectant women to keep as much as possible out of the way of such objects, and to preserve body and mind in a state of health, which will lessen the fear of being affected by such occurrences, and endeavor to direct the attention as much as possible to pleasing subjects, as it must be evident that *brooding over such unpleasant impressions* can scarcely fail of being both physically and mentally injurious."

MENTAL EMOTIONS, DESPONDENCY.—In some cases, and especially with delicate, sensitive ladies, and more commonly with first children, there is a great desponding of mind, dread of the future, and fear of approaching death. Some women, who in general have a fine flow of spirits, are particularly depressed and gloomy during this period, and with others there is this depression during the period of nursing. When it occurs early during gestation, it usually passes off before delivery, and is in no case to be considered as an unfavorable indication, and is in general without injury to the physical health.

TREATMENT.—Our method of treatment will do much to remove or mitigate it. When this condition is attended with some febrile movement, fullness of the head, or heat of the hands, the Specific No. ONE, two pellets taken dry on the tongue morning and at night, will be sufficient to remove it. When it is attended with morning sickness, the Specific No. TEN may be taken at night, and the No. TWENTY-NINE, two pellets in the morning, will afford relief to both affections. When there is excessive dejection and great lassitude, the No. THIRTY-FIVE may be given, two pellets at a time, three times per day. These remedies will usually be found quite adequate for the removal of any difficulties of this nature.

## MENSTRUATION DURING PREGNANCY.

Usually, with the commencement of pregnancy, menstruation ceases. In some cases, however, it may continue in some degree during the period of gestation, especially the first two or three months. It should not be considered as a disease, strictly speaking, yet it is one of those abnormal conditions which require attention, and should be remedied at the earliest moment.

TREATMENT.—Two pellets of the Specific No. TEN, taken

at night, and the same quantity of No. THIRTY-FIVE each morning, will, in general, arrest the discharge. Should the discharge be attended with cramps, pain, or bearing down, the Specific No. THIRTY-ONE should be taken in preference, two pellets every two, three or four hours, according to the urgency of the case, until relieved. Should the discharge again appear the subsequent month, the same treatment should be pursued, and so continue so long as is required.

## MORNING SICKNESS.

Nausea, vomiting, heartburn, constituting what is usually termed morning sickness, is one of the frequent and annoying accompaniments of pregnancy. In some cases these symptoms appear immediately, or soon after conception, but in most cases at about the sixth week. The most decided symptoms occur in the morning soon after rising, though in many cases they continue all through the day and are quite marked in the afternoon. The usual symptoms are nausea, qualmishness, then vomiting; sometimes only a single retching, at others severe and oft-repeated vomitings, with constant loss of appetite, and heartburn. In general these symptoms disappear soon after quickening, about the fourth month, but in others they attend and annoy during the entire period. In some cases these symptoms form but a trifling annoyance, scarcely noticeable, at others they form a most distressing and painful attendant of this interesting period. In some cases the suffering has been so terrible, and the remedies of old school medicine so fruitless, that premature delivery has been resorted to. Our treatment, fortunately, contemplates no such serious alternatives, as in general, all the serious symptoms, and even the inconveniences of the period are promptly relieved.

TREATMENT.—The Specific No. TWENTY-NINE is very

generally efficient. Take two pellets dry on the tongue at night on retiring, and in the morning *before* rising, and again at mid-day if needful. In some severe cases it may be better to dissolve six or eight pellets in as many spoonfuls of water, and of this take a spoonful every two hours during the waking hours. In some extreme cases, when the nausea and vomiting is excessive, the Specific No. SIX may be taken in the same manner as above indicated. If constipation, No. TEN at night and the No. TWENTY-NINE in the morning, two pellets.

## CONSTIPATION.

Constipation, more or less marked, is a very common attendant of pregnancy. If persons are habitually of constipated habit, it becomes more decided during this period. Much may be done to obviate this difficulty by active exercise in the open air, avoiding indigestible food, coffee, or other stimulating liquids, and by using such articles of food as are of a relaxing nature. Should medicine be required, the use of the Specific No. TEN, two pellets dissolved in water and taken night and morning, will be found sufficient. In some cases the Specific No. TWENTY-NINE, two pellets at night, and the No. TEN in the morning, will answer the purpose better. Enemas of tepid water may be resorted to if necessary.

## DIARRHŒA.

In some cases, diarrhœa more or less decided, or in occasional attacks, occurs during pregnancy, and especially in the latter stages, should demand attention. The usual remedies for this disease, as mentioned in the chapter on that subject, will be found efficient. Generally a few doses of the Specific No. FOUR, two pellets taken dry, and repeated after every stool, will be sufficient to arrest the difficulty. If the discharges are very loose and watery, the Specific No. SIX may be more appropriate.

## DYSURIA.

Difficulty in passing the water is not of unfrequent occurrence with pregnant women. It is attended with frequent inclination to pass water, accompanied with smarting, scalding, or burning, or there may be frequent urging with only scanty, painful discharge, approaching strangury. It will be promptly remedied by taking the Specific No. THIRTY, two pellets at a time, and repeated every two or three hours, until relieved. No. ELEVEN is sometimes equally serviceable.

## FAINTING AND HYSTERIA.

Delicate, sensitive, or nervous women, are sometimes attacked with turns of fainting during pregnancy. They are generally without serious annoyance, and pass over readily. Plenty of exercise in the open air, and attention to proper rules of diet and regimen, are the best preventatives against this affection; but in cases where these prove insufficient, we should endeavor to ascertain and remove the cause. Tight lacing, warm rooms, the free use of coffee or other stimulants may be the exciting cause, and their simple removal will prove efficient. Should an attack not inmediately pass off, loosening the dress, removal to the fresh air, and sprinkling the face with cold water, are the most judicious means of revival. The Specific No. THREE will at once quiet the nervous excitability of the system, and may be given in portions of two pellets, repeated hourly, if occasion requires. To prevent the recurrence of similar attacks, especially if the patient be of full or plethoric habit, the Specific No. THIRTY-FIVE may be given, two pellets night and morning. These remedies will rarely fail to afford the desired relief.

## TOOTHACHE.

This is a very frequent and annoying affection in the earlier months of pregnancy, and is sometimes one of its earliest indications. It is generally due to some constitutional taint in the system, and is brought into activity in this direction by the new action set up in the organization. It deserves attention, not only as a relief from the annoyance of suffering, but as a means of repressing the original dyscrasia of the system, and thus preventing even more serious manifestations. It is very injudicious for ladies under such circumstances, to hasten to a dentist and have one or several sound teeth extracted, to relieve what is simply a neurosis, excited by the transient condition of the system. It frequently occurs in sound teeth, and when one or more is extracted, may readily appear or seem to attack others, so that the loss of the teeth, and the suffering of having them extracted, may fail to relieve the pain. A little patience, and the use of the appropriate medicines, will not only relieve the pain and suffering, but also save the teeth.

TREATMENT.—As the affection is constitutional, quite a number of remedies may be appropriate, and merely local applications are often inefficient; nevertheless, when teeth have extensive cavities, filling them with cotton-wool saturated with HUMPHREYS' WITCH HAZEL, or holding a spoonful in the mouth, on the side where the tooth is, and wetting a cloth in the same and binding it on the face, are useful palliatives and often efficient in allaying the pain.

The Specific No. EIGHT may be first tried, two pellets dry, and administered every hour. Should relief not be afforded in some hours, give Specific No. THREE in the

16

same manner. Should there be throbbing in the teeth or face, No. ONE will be efficient. In very sensitive, nervous subjects, Specific No. ELEVEN has proved promptly curative. In full blooded, plethoric subjects, Specific No. THIRTY-FIVE has often cured. These remedies, or even others may be used in succession, or even in alternation, with success.

## SWELLED FACE.

Swelled face—tumefaction of the cheek—may arise from different causes. It is not unfrequently a result of toothache, the cheek beginning to swell as the pain in the teeth subsides. In this case it generally subsides by merely continuing the remedy which has been used to relieve the toothache. In other cases, binding up the face with a compress wet with WITCH HAZEL, and the use of Specifics No. ONE and No. ELEVEN, given in doses of two pellets, and repeated every two hours in alternation, will prove efficient.

## VARICES—SWELLED VEINS.

It not unfrequently occurs in the later months of gestation, that some women suffer from distention and enlargement of the veins of the thighs, lower abdomen, and of other parts. The veins in these situations become enlarged, blue and turgid, inducing sometimes pain and much inconvenience. They are in part occasioned by the pressure of the gravid uterus upon the blood vessels, thus obstructing the circulation, and in part from constitutional weakness of the individual, reflected upon the venous circulation. Unless relieved, the varices are liable to remain even after the occasioning cause has disappeared, and to give serious inconvenience in after life. They are much increased by the use of stimulants, which should, under such circumstances, be avoided, as well as an indolent habit of life.

TREATMENT.—A reasonable amount of exercise should be enjoined, and the parts affected should be bathed morning and night with WITCH HAZEL. Half a teaspoonful of the WITCH HAZEL should be taken internally three times per day. See also the treatment of *Varicose Veins.*

## PAINS IN THE BACK—LUMBO-SACRAL PAINS.

Some women suffer during pregnancy from pains in the lower part of the back, sometimes proving quite distressing, especially when they occur at night, and thereby disturb sleep. They are generally described as an aching, or a dull, heavy, dragging pressure, as if from a weight resting upon the affected part. They will usually be relieved by the use of the Specific No. FIFTEEN, two pellets three or four times per day. Sometimes they are associated with PILES, in which case the Specific No. SEVENTEEN may prove the more efficient remedy, and may be given as above, or may even be given in alternation with the No. FIFTEEN. Usually two pellets of No. TEN at night, and of No. FIFTEEN each morning, will afford satisfactory relief.

## MISCARRIAGE.

Miscarriage may occur at any period between the first and seventh month, but in the large proportion of cases, it occurs about the third or beginning of the fourth month. When it takes place *before* or *about* this period, it is frequently attended with but comparatively little pain or danger, yet frequent miscarriages at this period, from the great discharges that take place, tend to undermine the strength and constitution of the patient, and not unfrequently produce as a result, barrenness or severe chronic disease. When miscarriage occurs at a more advanced period, it assumes a very serious complexion, and is often attended with a considerable degree of peril to the sufferer. Women who have once suffered from the occurrence of a miscarriage, are exceedingly liable to its recurrence, and this liability is increased with every subsequent miscarriage, so that in a comparatively short period, a condition is induced which renders it exceedingly difficult for the womb to retain the fœtus up to the full term, resulting in a very intractable form of sterility.

The premonitory and accompanying symptoms of miscarriage vary much in their nature; sometimes a discharge of blood occurs which is very profuse, and at others moderate or even inconsiderable; the pains in some instances are severe and protracted, and at others comparatively slight and of short duration.

*Sudden mental emotions,* or *great physical exertion,* mechanical injuries, such as shocks, blows, or falls, a *luxurious mode of life,* fashionable habits or dissipations, powerful aperients, *neglecting to take air or exercise,* are some of the more common exciting causes of the affection, and to this should be added, that the predisposition is strong in the *highly plethoric,* and those of *delicate* and *nervous habits.* An abnormal condition of the system is doubtless the predisposing cause.

Miscarriage is generally attended by the majority of the following symptoms: A sensation of chill, followed by fever, with more or less bearing down, particularly when occuring late in pregnancy; also *severe pains in the abdomen, drawing or cutting pains in the loins,* or pains often bearing a close resemblance to those of labor; discharge of viscid mucus and blood, sometimes of *bright red* blood, not unfrequently mixed with coagula, at other times *dark* and clotted blood, followed by emissions of serous fluid. The miscarriage generally occurs during this discharge, which occasionally continues, if not checked, to flow for some hours, often placing the sufferer in considerable jeopardy. When the pains increase in intensity, and the muscular contractions become established with their regular throes and efforts to dilate the mouth of the womb, miscarriage is almost inevitable.

Treatment.—In cases where a woman has had one or more miscarriages, it is evident that a predisposition to this accident exists, and more than usual care should be exercised to prevent a similar result, and such persons should especially avoid all the exciting causes which have been above mentioned. But beside these prudential considerations in habits, labor and exercise, proper medicine may be taken to allay or remove that morbid irritability of the uterus, which lays at the foundation of the difficulty. To this end the Specific No. Eleven, simply two pellets taken every other night, and continued along during the period mentioned, from the second to the fourth month, will prove efficacious. Sometimes the occasional use of *Sabina,* sixth dilution, or of *Secale,* same dilution, given at intervals of six or eight days, will produce a similar result.

When the symptoms indicating an impending miscarriage have made their appearance, such as: A *slight show,* sensation of dull, heavy pressure in the back or loins, pains in the lower abdomen, bearing down or dragging, the patient should at once retire to her room, assume the recumbent posture, or in some cases go to bed and sleep with but slight covering; the apartment should be kept cool, and every method be employed to ensure perfect tranquillity of mind. The diet should be light, and warm or stimulating drinks be generally avoided. If the misfortune has proved unavoidable, or has accidentally taken place before assistance has been sought, the patient ought still to remain quiet a few days, lest a fresh discharge should be brought on from too early getting up or going about. When the first symptoms mentioned above are perceived, four pellets of Specific No. ELEVEN should be taken dry on the tongue, and perfect rest and quiet enjoined. If not better in an hour, take the same quantity of Specific No. THREE, and continue these two medicines in alternation, at intervals of one, two or three hours, according to circumstances, always taking care to diminish the frequency of doses as the symptoms diminish or disappear.

Should the miscarriage have occurred, or become inevitable from the great loss of blood, four pellets of Specific No. TWENTY-FOUR, given every half, or even every quarter of an hour, will be among the best means to arrest the flow, and relieve the faintness, exhaustion, and debility in consequence of the hemorrhage. The same medicine, No. TWENTY-FOUR, given four times per day, best relieves the exhaustion and debility resulting from such hemorrhage or accident. In extreme cases, when the excessive hemorrhage, occurring at later periods of pregnancy, produce faintness, great exhaustion, or threaten life from their excess or long continuance, the use of POND'S EXTRACT, half a teaspoonful, repeated every half hour at first, and then every one or two hours, according to circumstances, acts like magic, arrests the frightful flow, and recalls the waning spark.

## TREATMENT BEFORE PARTURITION.

PREPARATION OF THE BREASTS.—Young mothers frequently find great difficulty in suckling their children, resulting from some organic defect, or imperfect development of the nipple. In many instances the structure of the breasts is disorganized, from an ignorant nurse having compressed them in infancy, under the idea of such a process being needful for the expulsion of some matter in the breast of the child, a vulgar error, against which mothers should be particularly watchful. Inability to nurse is also liable to occur from the pressure of stays in after life, by which the cuticle is rendered so tender as to preclude nursing. In almost every case a preparation of the breasts is necessary some weeks before delivery, in order to prepare them for their future office.

The first two instances, organic defect or an undeveloped nipple, may be beyond the power of art. If suckling be attempted, induration of the nipple and mamma ensues, attended with severe suffering. If, however, a simple tenderness of the epidermis exists, the evil will be much alleviated by bathing the nipples in brandy each morning and night for several weeks before delivery. Another difficulty frequently accompanying this state, is a shortness or retraction of the nipple, so that the infant cannot take hold of it, which also is frequently a cause of the first, from the frequent ineffectual efforts of the infant to suck, injuring the part. In this case, appropriate shields of rubber or wood may be applied, to accustom the nipple to elongate and protrude, so as to present a sufficient hold for the infant when the period for suckling arrives, and then the efforts of the child will still further contribute to the same object. In this case also, bathing as before mentioned, with brandy, will tend to correct any tenderness of the skin, and prevent subsequent excoriation.

Remedies Before Labor.—Many things have been recommended before labor, and among them blood-letting and aperient medicines, with a view of preparing the system for the important function. But better judgment and experience has discarded them as being in no wise necessary, but often injurious, tending to impair the energies of the system, and to place the system in an abnormal state of irritation and excitement. Where an evidently plethoric state exists, with fullness of the head and person generally, four pellets of Specific No. ONE, repeated daily, or even more frequently if the occasion demands, will be found fully sufficient for the purpose, and will serve a far better purpose than bleeding or aperients.

A movement of the bowels previous to delivery is desirable, and may be obtained by a simple enema of warm water, to which may be added, if the simple warm water should prove insufficient, a large spoonful of oil, in a second enema.

FALSE PAINS.—In some cases real labor is preceded for a few hours, and indeed in others several days or even weeks, by what are known as *false pains.* They are the result of congestion of the organs involved, and result from errors in regimen, emotions of the mind, effects of a chill in the abdomen, or other exciting causes. They differ chiefly from labor pains, *in the irregularity of their recurrence, in being unconnected with uterine contractions, are chiefly confined to the abdomen, with sensibility to touch and movement, and in not increasing in intensity as they return.* Occasionally, from their close resemblance, it is quite difficult to discriminate between them and real labor pains, and in such instances we must be guided chiefly by the period of gestation, and our proper and safe mode is to endeavor to control them, if they occur at a period some week or two before the proper time for labor, and mitigate the sufferings of the patient, as, if they are permitted to go on unchecked, they may continue until the time of delivery, rendering the labor more painful, exhausting, and tedious. Proper medication will, in general, either arrest them, or convert them into true labor pains.

TREATMENT.—Generally a few doses of Specific No. ONE, four pellets, repeated at intervals of one or two hours, will be found sufficient. Should, however, the result not be satisfactory, administer Specific No. ELEVEN in the same manner, or give the Specific No. THREE, if the patient should be very nervous or excitable.

## PARTURITION.

Natural labor takes place at the end of the ninth month of pregnancy, or two hundred and seventy days from the period of conception. Counting six weeks to the usual appearance of morning sickness, and four months to the period of quickening, and nine months from the last menstruation, the period of labor may be looked for with tolerable certainty. The pains accompanying uterine contractions are regular and effective, and the entire process does not continue beyond twenty-four hours, rarely above twelve, and quite frequently not longer than four or six. Were it not that acquired habits often derange or distort the natural and symmetrical provisions of nature, habits that weaken and enervate, and customs that distort and derange, either acquired or transmitted, parturition would be comparatively free from pain and almost free from danger.

## TEDIOUS LABORS.

When labor is protracted beyond the period above mentioned, or is attended with an excessive degree of suffering, which is the more liable to occur when the woman is of slender form, and of highly nervous and sensitive habit, it is proper to avail ourselves of all the resources of art, to mitigate her sufferings.

Thus, if the pains seem to be ineffective, the face red and flushed, and the patient distressed, out of proportion to the effectiveness of the pains, give four pellets of the Specific No. ONE, and repeat it in an hour if not relieved.

If the pains are what are called wrangling, in the abdomen or lower extremities, and not from the back, drawing down forward, give the No. ELEVEN in the same manner.

If the patient is very nervous, excitable, and the pains slight or inefficient, even with some tendency to cramps of the extremities, give the Specific No. THREE, four pellets every half hour, and repeat it until these symptoms yield, and the pains become strong and expulsive.

## CRAMPS AND CONVULSIONS.

In complicated labors we sometimes have spasmodic pains as indicated above, which do but little towards advancing the labor, and in rare cases, severe cramps, or even convulsions. These accidents are of serious import, and should be carefully guarded against, in cases where their indications exist. The Specific No. THREE should be given, four pellets dry on the tongue, and repeated every half hour, or hour, so long as extreme nervousness and excitability of the patient continues. Should this prove ineffective, and the excitement of the patient still continue, notwithstanding its use, and the very essential procedure of keeping the room quiet, and exciting persons or things as far removed as possible, or in case actual cramps or convulsions have supervened, give the Specific No. THIRTY-THREE, four pellets at once, and repeat it every hour until the danger is removed.

## TREATMENT AFTER DELIVERY.

Immediately after delivery, and the proper adjustment of the bed, the woman should be left to the undisturbed rest and repose which are the great restoratives of nature. Everything which tends to excite the patient—noise, light, talking, or excitement of any kind—should be avoided, and the patient be quietly allowed to rest for some hours; yet it is commendable to see that the discharges are not excessive, and that the pulse is not sinking. An hour or two of good quiet rest will do more to restore, than tea, stimulants, or food at this time. Should the patient be kept from sleeping, from excitement, give four pellets of Specific No. THREE, which will soon allay it, and serve also to stimulate the natural contractions of the womb. In the event of too profuse discharge, or even flooding, the No. THREE may be given, four pellets every half hour, or should there be faintness, or very profuse flow, a half teaspoonful of WITCH HAZEL may at once be resorted to, and repeated every half hour until it is controlled.

The patient should mostly keep her bed for the first eight days; after four or six days, if she feels strong and so desires, she may be permitted to sit up a short period daily, to have her bed made and aired. It is important for the womb to reduce itself and recover its natural position; that the woman be kept at rest, and in a recumbent posture for the eight or fourteen days, and careful attention to this advice will prevent much of infirmity, debility, and after disease. The diet should be of light and easily-digested food, avoiding all stimulants or exciting beverages, and being guided in quantity by the desires of the patient, bearing in mind that for the first few days, nature calls for but little nourishment, and that if given when the patient does not desire it, it will be more liable to be injurious then beneficial. All stimulating or very nutritious food must be avoided the first few days.

For the constipation, which is the natural result of delivery, nothing should be done at first, as it is altogether a proper and salutary condition, time being required for the organs to regain their natural tone and position, which should not be interfered with by aperients. If after four or six days the bowels should not move spontaneously, an injection of warm water may be administered, and assisted by four pellets of Specific No. TEN, given at night, and these may be repeated, if necessary, until natural evacuations are established.

SUPPRESSED OR SCANTY SECRETION OF MILK.—It is of importance that the processes of nature follow in proper order, and with due regularity, and hence, it is proper to correct, so far as in our power, any important deviation. Sometimes the proper secretion of milk is prevented by undue heat, distention, excessive or undue vitality of the breasts. In such cases, a few doses of Specific No. ONE, four pellets given at intervals of four hours, will allay the heat and distention, and the secretion will proceed with regularity. If, however, the secretion seems to fail from a want of secretory power in the gland itself, the use of Specific No. ELEVEN, given in like manner, will promote the natural flow.

## MILK FEVER.

The secretion of milk in considerable quantities is often preceded or accompanied with a general febrile movement of the system, which is known by the term of *milk fever*. It is known by thirst, slight shivering and heat, terminating in mild perspiration; the pulse is quickened, and sometimes variable; at times frequent, or soft and regular. Sometimes there is drawing pain in the back, extending to the breast, bad taste in the mouth, oppressed respiration, anxiety and headache, the exacerbation comes on towards evening, with perspiration towards morning, and temporary relief or termination of the attack, which not unfrequently returns the following day, but rarely rises to such a hight as to indicate danger. Nature herself, if not disturbed by injudicious treatment, in most cases restores the proper equilibrium. When the milk secretion is established, and the lochial discharge resumes its wonted course, the derangement generally ceases. Should, however, the affection become established, we may apprehend the setting in of puerperal fever.

The indications above mentioned call for the Specific No. ONE, which may best be given by dissolving twelve pellets in six spoonfuls of water, of which one may be given every hour at first, and then at intervals of two hours, until the fever quite disappears, and the normal secretions are established.

## LOCHIAL DISCHARGE.

This discharge continues, usually, from nine to fourteen days, but varies considerably in different women, sometimes being but slight, at others, copious and continuing for a long time. Its deviations require attention. If it becomes suppressed, or thin, pale, and prematurely scanty, Specific No. ELEVEN should be given, four pellets every two or three hours. If pain and fever attend the diminution or suppression, No. ONE should be given in water, four pellets every hour, until this condition is removed. If it is too free, or remains full or high-colored after nine days, Specific No. TWENTY-FOUR should be given, four pellets three times per day.

## DIARRHŒA DURING CONFINEMENT.

Diarrhœa at this period may be considered as exceedingly prejudicial, and always demands attention. It will usually be removed by the use of Specific No. FOUR, of which four pellets may be taken after every stool. Thus the frequency of the stools will be the measure of the frequency of the doses. Of course the diet should be so regulated as to remove any occasioning cause in that source. *See Diarrhœa.*

## FALLING OUT OF THE HAIR.

Not unfrequently, and especially in feeble or debilitated constitutions, the hair falls out, during or soon after the period of confinement. If the patient has become debilitated in consequence of flooding, or the excessive drains upon the system, the evil will be corrected by the use of Specific No. Twenty-four, taking four pellets three times per day. If the cause is not so apparent, and must be sought for in some inherent delicacy of the constitution, the use of Specifics No. Thirty-five, and No. Twenty-nine, giving four pellets of the former in the morning, and the latter at night. Care should be taken in dressing the hair during this condition of the scalp, not to comb or brush it too harshly, as you may thus pull out large quantities of hair that a more appropriate management would have preserved.

## LEUCORRHŒA AFTER PARTURITION.

This appears to be at first only an extension of the natural discharges in consequence of the relaxation of the uterine economy, at the beginning mild and inocuous, but gradually assuming an acrid or morbid condition, producing sensibility and excoriation. It is sometimes very obstinate and often troublesome. Specifics No. Twelve and Eleven are the proper remedies. Give of the first, four pellets morning and night for a week. If not controlled, give No. Eleven in the same manner. When it depends upon a scrofulous taint in the system, the No. Twenty-two will be useful. Injections of Witch Hazel and water, in the proportion of one part of the same and two parts of water, administered morning and night, are of the utmost possible value in arresting such discharges, stimulating contractions, and giving tone and vigor to the organs.

## INTERNAL SWELLING AND PROLAPSUS.

A swelling of interior organs is frequently the result of difficult labor, and is often found complicated with uterine or vaginal prolapsus. The use of **WITCH HAZEL** externally as a lavement, and as an injection prepared as above, one part of the same to two of water, is sovereign in all similar cases, and may be administered two or three times per day. At the same time, Specific No. THIRTY-FIVE, four pellets, may be given three times per day.

## INFLAMMATION OF THE WOMB—MITRITIS.

The more constant symptoms of this very serious affection, are: Fever, pain, continuous burning or shooting in the lower abdominal region, accompanied with a sensation of weight; soreness or tenderness of that region on pressure or movement. The abdomen becomes hot, and gradually tumefied, the secretion of lochia and milk diminished or arrested, likewise the urine and feces. It is usually caused by severe, unnatural or protracted labors, or by harsh manual interference during labor, or may result from retained placenta or clots, or mental emotions, chill, etc. In a less active form, it may occur in women who have never borne children, as the result of chill, cold feet, inflammation of neighboring organs, external injuries, etc.

The Specific No. ONE should be given, twelve pellets dissolved in six large spoonfuls of water, of which one should be given every hour, and this medication continued with entire rest and quiet until the power of the disease is broken, and the normal discharges re-established.

## EXCORIATION OF THE NIPPLES.

If the nipples have been properly prepared for their office by frequent bathing with brandy, WITCH HAZEL, or other hardening preparations, there will be less liability of excoriation; nevertheless, it sometimes appears, notwithstanding, owing to some dyscrasia of the system. The nipples become sore, excoriated or cracked, and bleed, and are exquisitely painful at every attempt of the child to nurse.

TREATMENT.—From the first, after every nursing, the nipples should be carefully moistened with WITCH HAZEL, diluted one half with water, and, after being thus thoroughly moistened, should be carefully dried with a soft cloth or fine lint, and this process should be constantly repeated after nursing. In some cases a soft rubber shield can be worn to advantage, but to be effective, it must fit nicely, and be worn easily. Internally, the Specific No. THREE should be given, four pellets three times per day, to remove any constitutional impediment to the healing. In cases where these remedies remain ineffectual, resort may be had to a dose of four pellets of Specific No. TWENTY-TWO, at night, while the No. THREE is given morning and at noon, and so continue for some days.

## INFLAMMATION OF THE BREASTS—GATHERED BREAST.

A very formidable and painful affection is what is known as ague in the breast, or gathered breasts. It commences with a chill, to which some degree of fever is soon associated, and the breast, or some portion of it becomes tumefied, swelled, sensitive and painful, with an erysipelatous swelling and redness extending over some portion of the surface. In case the inflammation is not early arrested, suppuration takes place, the swelling points, and the abscess must be opened and pus discharged, or it will of itself open, causing a much more extensive disorganization and discharge, and a disfiguring cicatrix.

TREATMENT.—Specific No. ONE should be given at once, twelve pellets dissolved in six dessert spoonfuls of water, and of this a large spoonful should be given every hour for the first twelve hours, and then every two hours, until the inflammation subsides. Advantage will also be derived from the application of a cloth, several folds of which have been saturated with WITCH HAZEL, and applied well over the part or breast, and the whole covered with flannel, so as to protect the clothing and person from moisture, and the application may be removed as often as it gets hot or dry.

If the inflammation has progressed so far that suppuration cannot be arrested, or has already taken place, the use of Specific No. TWENTY-TWO, four pellets every three hours, will be the best medicine to promote that object, and at the same time to limit its extension. It is likewise the best medicine to limit the suppurative process, and heal the wound after the abscess has been opened.

## WEAKNESS OR PERSPIRATION DURING CONFINEMENT.

Sometimes there remains an excessive degree of debility after delivery, continuing several weeks beyond the usual period, and in consequence the patient sweats easily during any effort, or on going to sleep. This condition of weakness, indicating an exhausted or enfeebled vitality, is best met by Specific No. TWENTY-FOUR, of which two pellets may be given dry, four times per day, with advantage, or simply at night, two pellets, if there is merely too free perspiration at night, or on sleeping.

## TREATMENT OF INFANTS.

Homeopathy possesses many advantages in the treatment of the diseases of children and infants. The first manifestations of morbid action are thus met in their formative stage, and not only are they crushed in the bud, but the tendency thereto is eradicated from the system. Constitutional tendencies to disease are thus destroyed, and the entire development is symmetrical and happy. On the contrary, when the diseases of infancy and early childhood are met by the pernicious drugs so much in vogue in the old school of medicine, not only are the diseases themselves not eradicated from the system, but drug action is often set up, false, perverted or morbid action is engendered, and the germs of what become life-long maladies are thus unwisely planted. Thousands of illy-developed, misanthropic, and unhappily constituted persons, owe their life-long infirmities to the injudicious use of drugs or crude medicines, given with the best intentions during their infancy.

## TREATMENT AFTER BIRTH.

Immediately after the separation of the cord, the child should be wrapped in a soft flannel, which has been carefully warmed, and be laid upon its *left* side. After the mother has been cared for, the child should be washed with tepid water, with a soft cloth, care being taken not to continue the first washing too long, not to rub the child, nor to apply soap, as the skin is very delicate and tender, and the entire organism unaccustomed to cold, or to rough usage. After washing, dry the infant immediately, by taking up the moisture with a soft, warm cloth, rather than by rubbing, always avoiding the risk of the child becoming chilled or taking cold. Nor should infants be swathed or overburdened with a superfluity of clothes, a source of not unfrequent deformity and weakness.

SWELLING OF THE HEAD very commonly appears in infants to some extent, and sometimes, indeed, a large tumor appears, which seems very formidable, and excites apprehension. This swelling generally disappears of itself after a few days. Should it be considerable, wetting the head with WITCH HAZEL, diluted one-half with tepid water, will rapidly promote the absorption of the tumor. Should there be a swelling which seems to contain fluid over the fontanel or large opening on the head, one pellet of Specific No. TWENTY-TWO will hasten its removal.

EXPULSION OF THE MECONIUM is best effected by the natural milk of the mother, which, at its first appearance after delivery, has the precise qualities adapted to that purpose. Hence, so soon as the child begins to desire food, and the mother has recovered sufficient strength to permit it, say from eight to twelve hours after birth, the child may be applied to the breast. Should it get but a trifle, even that will be of benefit to the child, and the effort will stimulate the secretion, so that after a few times it will become established. Its gradual appearance is better than to have it come in a flood, with fever after two or more days. On no account should drugs or domestic herb teas be given to the child to promote this object. A spoonful of sweetened water from time to time will be much better, or even an injection of equal parts of pure sweet oil and water.

THE DIET OF THE NURSE should be simple, easily digested, and a due proportion of vegetable and animal food. That which is too highly concentrated or stimulating may be injurious, by causing the milk to become too rich and unsuited to the delicate digestion of the infant. In some rare cases, wine, ale, or even porter, may be used to promote the secretion, and sustain the strength of the nurse. But in more cases evil is done than good, and in general the resort to the use of stimulants should be avoided. and the system should be sustained by those best purveyors of nature, quiet, avoidance of fatigue, anxiety, good food and sufficient sleep.

SUPPLEMENTARY DIET OF INFANTS.—The best and most natural food is the milk of the mother. Even if this only in part supplies the want of the child, it is better to retain even this, as in case of sickness of the infant, it furnishes a precious reserve to be supplied in no other way. *Cows' milk* is the most usual substitute, and should at first be diluted by adding one-third of water, and slightly sweetened. If milk is to remain some time during warm weather, it should be first heated to prevent too rapid change. Great care should be taken that the nursing bottle be *perfectly clean* and sweet, and food which has been standing, or is in danger of having deteriorated, must on no account be given. Better make that which you know to be sweet and fresh, than to assume a risk. After some weeks the milk may be given without water, and as the first teeth appear, about the fourth or sixth month, the diet should become more varied and liberal; a well made panada, diluted milk, sweetened and thickened with a small quantity of arrowroot, sago or rusk, may be given with advantage. So barley-water, well-boiled gruel, weak chicken-tea or beef-tea, may be resorted to, taking care to give that on which the child seems to thrive best. Gradually, as the teeth appear, the child may be given the usual food from the table, and in such quantities, and in such form, as the organism seems to require.

WEANING.—The length of time a child should nurse, depends upon many considerations, such as: The health of the child, of the mother, and the season of the year, and the facility of substituting an appropriate diet. In general, a child should be nursed from nine to fifteen months. If care be taken to gradually substitute a proper diet, a child will gradually wean itself before that period. The child had better not be weaned suddenly, but gradually, and in proportion as the teeth appear. With the full development of the teeth, the organism is generally prepared to thrive without the aid of the breast. Weaning during the hot season is hazardous, from the liability to diarrhœas, or the usual summer complaints.

## DISEASES OF INFANTS.

INFLAMMATION OF THE EYES of new-born infants may arise from sudden exposure to the strong glare of daylight. If the eyes look red, and shrink from the light, or are tearful, watery, dissolve a single pellet of Specific No. ONE in a spoonful of water, and give of this a few drops once per day for two or three days. If not cured, give a single pellet of No. EIGHTEEN in the same manner, keeping the child's eyes free from the irritation of all bright light.

COLD IN THE HEAD usually takes the form of obstruction of the nose, impeding the action of suckling, and causing the infant to release the nipple, and rendering it irritable and fretful. If the nose is dry within, we may imitate the natural secretion by applying a little almond oil or cream on a feather to the interior of the nostril. Usually the Specific No. THREE, one pellet given three times per day, will remove the difficulty. If it fails, give the No. NINETEEN in the same manner. It may be given in water, or even dry in the mouth, after the child is some weeks old.

CRYING AND WAKEFULNESS OF INFANTS will, with proper care to the diet and regimen of the mother and child, be fully obviated by the use of Specific No. THREE. Of course the child must be properly changed, made comfortable and satisfied with food, and it must not be taking with its food from the mother the flatulent food or exciting drinks, coffee, strong tea, or other stimulants which she imbibes. These conditions met, the No. THREE will afford quiet, refreshing sleep and rest, and freedom from the colic and cries so common in the nursery. Of course all drops, soothing syrups, or anodynes must be banished.

REGURGITATIONS OF FOOD.—Children often in nursing overload themselves with milk, and as a salutary provision, they regurgitate or throw up a portion of it. No interference is required in such cases. But where all, or a large portion of the food taken is thrown up again, or the regurgitated matter is sour, and is followed by mucus or watery fluid, or the children are sick, or appear nauseated, medical interference is desirable. In such cases an occasional pellet of Specific No. TEN will correct the action of the stomach. Should there be nausea or actual vomiting, Specific No. SIX, given as above, will be better. It may be given dissolved in a spoonful of water, or even dry to somewhat older children.

MILK CRUSTS—ERUPTIONS.—A scurvy eruption sometimes appear upon the hairy scalp, which in places becomes brownish bran-like. The application of a drop or two of nice sweet-oil, with the gentle aid of a soft brush or fine comb soon removes it, care being taken not to injure the surface. Meantime a pellet of Specific No. FOURTEEN, given at night for a few days, will arrest the tendency to its production.

MILK CRUSTS appear in the form of an eruption of small, whitish vesicles, appearing in clusters upon a reddish base, coming first upon the face, cheeks and forehead, thence extending to other parts. The lymph contained in these vesicles soon becomes yellow or dark, and bursting from thin yellow crusts. There is considerable redness, swelling, itching, and irritation, causing the child to become restless and fretful, continually rubbing the parts, which increases the discharge, until the crusts become thickened, sometimes covering the entire face, the nose and eyes only remaining free. The eyes and lids, and the glands of face and neck and abdomen, sometimes become involved, and marasmus may supervene. For these cases the Specific

No. FOURTEEN, one pellet for infants, or two for children over one year of age, may be given morning, noon, and at night, each dissolved in a spoonful of water. If the itching is severe, causing restlessness and fretfulness, dissolve of Specific No. ONE, six pellets in as many spoonfuls of water, and of this give a spoonful every hour between the intermediate doses of No. FOURTEEN, and this No. ONE may be thus used as an intermediate remedy, so long as the itching and irritation continues. A trifle of sweet oil will at any time remove the crusts. But they had better fall off of themselves, and I advise to apply soap or water to them as seldom as the purposes of cleanliness will permit.

THRUSH OR APHTHÆ shows itself by the formation of small, isolated, round, white vesicles, which if not checked may run together, and present an ulcerated appearance, or form a thin, white crust, which lines the entire cavity of the mouth, and in severe cases involves the throat and entire alimentary canal. It is rarely dangerous or malignant, but occasions inconvenience besides pain and suffering, obstructing the child's nursing, and may be communicated to the nipples, causing excoriation, etc. It is often the result of imperfect ventilation, inattention to cleanliness, the nursing bottle not being kept perfectly clean and sweet, improper food, etc. Hence, infants brought up by hand, as it is termed, are more subject to the disease than others. A very weak solution of BORAX, applied to the mouth with a brush, is very generally useful. The Specific No. TWENTY-NINE, four pellets dissolved in as many spoonfuls of water, and given, a spoonful every four hours, will be found sufficient to remove the disease. When it exists in only a slighter degree, a single pellet given dry, morning and night, will be sufficient.

CONSTIPATION will rarely be troublesome among children properly nursed or nourished, and under Homeopathic regimen. But should the stools be too large, tardy, insufficient or obstructed, dissolve of Specific No. Ten, two pellets in two large spoonfuls of water, of which give one at night, and the other in the morning, and this may be continued until the dejections become natural. An enema of tepid water may occasionally be resorted to if necessary, or a suppository, consisting of a small slip of paper or linen, spirally twisted and well lubricated with oil, may be introduced by a gentle rotatory movement from time to time, until the medicine has remedied the irregularity.

Diarrhœa of Infants.—Diarrhœa, like constipation, is merely a symptom and hardly a disease. It is an indication of an irritable condition of the intestinal track, and may arise from various causes; bad food, cold, fright, use of aperient medicines, etc. The first element of a cure for diarrhœa of infants, is to carefully examine as to the quality and quantity of its food and care, and to see that these give no occasion for the difficulty. The use of Specific No. Three from time to time, for colic, crying, sleeplessness, or teething, will usually check any predisposition to diarrhœa, or it may be used for this purpose, giving to infants one pellet dry in the mouth after every loose or diarrhœic stool. Should this not prove sufficient, the Specific No. Four may be administered in the same manner, one pellet after every loose stool; thus the urgency of the symptom will be the measure of the repetition of the medicine.

Excoriations—Intertrigo.—Cleanliness is the best preventive; careful bathing, and taking special care that all the folds of the skin, such as the neck, groin, etc., be carefully wiped dry with lint or soft cloth. The Specific No. Three is here also appropriate, to remove any tendencies to these excoriations, and may be given for such purpose, one pellet three times per day.

Derangements during Teething. The production of teeth, like other evolutions of the system, is attended with some degree of constitutional disturbance. In most cases and under Homeopathic regimen, these derangements are slight and easily removed, in others they may be more serious. Should there be, as is more frequently the case, RESTLESSNESS, WORRYING, sleeplessness, and tardy appearance of the teeth, the No. THREE is the proper Specific, and may be given one pellet dry in the mouth every hour or two hours, according to the urgency of the case. If diarrhœa sets in and becomes troublesome—remembering that a slight looseness of the bowels during this period is not prejudicial—it may be controlled by the Specific No. FOUR, one pellet after every loose stool. Should there be fever or heat of the head, crying and worrying, or drowsiness, have resource at once to the No. ONE, of which dissolve six pellets in twelve spoonfuls of water, and of this give a teaspoonful every hour until the fever, restlessness, or drowsiness has passed away.

CONVULSIONS OF INFANTS.—Infants are peculiarly liable to convulsions. At that early period the brain is proportionally larger, the nervous organization more delicate, and the various evolutions through which it is passing render it more liable to spasmodic or convulsive attacks, than at a subsequent period of life. The usual causes are intestinal irritation from improper food, the irritation of teething, to which should also be added, hereditary predisposition in some families, all the children being subject to convulsions on very slight provocation, while in others such an occurrence is unknown. Where children are hot, feverish, either sleep too soundly, or are very restless, and *start suddenly* on dropping into a dose or at other times, the access of convulsions is imminent and demands attention. First, the occasioning cause should be removed. If the child is constipated, or if there is reason to suppose the irritation is occasioned by indigestible, bad, or irritating food, give at once a full, free injection of tepid water. Should it not relieve the symptoms, or fail to produce a full movement of the bowels, repeat it after half an hour, and even again, until the result is obtained. Meantime, if there is heat or fever, hot head and hands, dissolve six pellets of Specific No. ONE in as many spoonfuls of water, and of this give a spoonful every half hour for two or three times, and then as the heat and fever abate, give every hour until relieved. Should there be not so much heat or fever, and the irritation of teething having been the cause, the Specific No. THREE, given as above, may be preferable to No. ONE. In case of a convulsion, but little can be done during the paroxysm, but so soon as practicable, the feet and legs should be immersed in warm water for several minutes, and then carefully wiped dry and wrapped in a warm cloth, and a cloth wet with cold water applied to the head, and the injection before mentioned be administered. In some cases the Specifics No. ONE and No. THREE, prepared as above, may be given alternately, a spoonful every hour, with advantage, and especially when the convulsions have been repeated, or the premonitions of them continue.

TO DESTROY A PREDISPOSITION to convulsions, or prevent the development of epilepsy, the Specific No. THIRTY-THREE may be given, one pellet every night, for three days, and the same of Specific No. THIRTY-FIVE each morning, and then every second night for some weeks, giving No. THIRTY-FIVE every morning.

## ATROPHY.

In cases where children do not seem to thrive, waste away, become emaciated, the tissue becoming atrophied, and a well marked marasmus occurs, any of the Specifics which meets these indications are efficient. Such a condition, indeed, very rarely happens under the Specific Homeopathic treatment. But should such a condition threaten, or have actually been developed, we should be guided in our choice of Specifics by the indications, thus: For enlarged abdomen, heat of the head, slow closing fontanelle, slow growth, give Specific No. THIRTY-FIVE. When there is constipated habit, tardy, insufficient evacuations, deranged stomach or pale stools, give the Specific No. TEN. If the glands become enlarged, with knots about the neck or under the arms, frequent boils, swellings, or tumors, give Specific No. TWENTY-THREE. If diarrhœa or constant tendency to loose bowels is present, give Specific No. FOUR. These remedies may usually be given in these cases, simply one pellet for infants three times per day, dry in the mouth.

## VACCINATION.

Much discussion has been had in late years as to the propriety or value of vaccination as a preventive for small-pox. The substance arrived at seems to be about this:—

I. That vaccination is a *measurable* protection against the small-pox; those who have been vaccinated being far less liable to the disease than those who have not been, but that this protection is by no means absolute or perfect.

II. That in vaccination there is always *some* danger of being thence infected by some chronic disease, communicated with the virus, or roused into activity by its introduction or dissemination in the system.

III. That could we know when an exposure or attack of small-pox was to take place, or were our remedial means what they ought to be, or as effective in this disease as we trust, ere long, they will be, it were better to run the risk of the disease, than the danger of impure or diseased-communicating virus.

IV. That in the present state of our knowledge, the danger of disease from vaccination is the lesser of the two, and that therefore we should vaccinate, taking care always that the virus employed is of the purest possible quality. It must not be taken from the squalid, the ill-fed or sickly, or those affected with any trace of skin disease, or scrofula, or those whose parents are suspected of any trace of syphilitic affection, or of scrofula. A strong, healthy child should be vaccinated about the fourth or fifth month, or at any time if the disease be prevalent, or the child has been exposed. The left arm at the upper third from the shoulder is the best point for the insertion of the virus, and during its working, a pellet of Specific No. FOURTEEN may be given every second or third night with a view to prevent any morbid development.

V. Re-vaccination is desirable, and the evidence is that the protection is greater where two or more scars exist, than where a single point is found.

# DISEASES OF VARIOUS ORGANS AND REGIONS.

## RHEUMATISM.

This very common, and sometimes quite obstinate disease, manifests itself mostly in two forms—the ACUTE or INFLAMMATORY, and the CHRONIC.

### ACUTE OR INFLAMMATORY RHEUMATISM.

It is usually brought on by exposure to cold, rough or damp weather, and especially to fatigue or labor during such exposure; also from sitting or standing in cold, damp places, or from sitting in a draught; sleeping in damp sheets or remaining long in wet clothes; exposure of any parts of the body to cold and moisture when other parts of the body are covered, or exposure when in a perspiration. There is probably, also a rheumatic diathesis or tendency, which may also be inherited. Sometimes it appears to arise from the suppression of an eruption, or the retrocession of measles, rash, or chicken-pox, or the suppression of some discharge like gonorrhœa or dysentery.

It generally commences with the usual signs of fever, associated with stiffness and lameness; chilliness and heat alternating; thirst and restlessness; coldness of the extremities, and usually constipation. After twelve or twenty-four hours the fever becomes continuous, the skin hot and dry; pulse quick, often 110 to 120 per minute. The stiffness and pain in the joints becomes more decided, with acute suffering especially on every attempt to move. The affected parts are usually red, swelled and extremely painful to the touch. Sometimes there is excessive pain without the redness or swelling; the pain is generally worse at night, and occasionally an acrid perspiration accompanies the disease.

The larger joints of the extremities are usually the seat of the disease. It is rarely confined to one, and sometimes nearly all, either simultaneously or in turn are affected so that often the patient can scarcely move hand or foot. Often the disease leaves one ankle, knee or wrist, and locates upon another, leaving the former comparatively free. During the course of the disease, complications with the heart are liable to arise from the rheumatic process having invaded that organ, a circumstance always undesirable and sometimes quite dangerous. It is more liable to occur when cold, chilling or severe applications such as blisters, are made to the affected joint, than under Homeopathic treatment. When there is a remission of the pain in the joints, followed by anxiety, jerking, feeble or rapid pulse, and acute pain in the region of the heart, there is reason to apprehend such a transition.

TREATMENT.—At the first symptoms of *acute rheumatism*, with soreness, lameness, and pain in the part, two pellets of Specific No. FIFTEEN should be taken every hour, dissolved in a spoonful of water, and the patient should remain in-doors, and keep quiet until relieved. If violent fever, heat and swelling of the part has already come on, as noticed above, indicating rheumatic fever, or a chill succeeded by heat, prepare Specific No ONE by dissolving eight pellets in half a glass of water, of which give a spoonful every hour for a day, and then prepare the No. FIFTEEN in the same manner, and take the two alternately every two hours. These should be continued from day to day, until the disease is broken up, preparing the medicine fresh every morning. Sometimes applications of cloths wrung out of tepid water, and laid on the part, are very soothing. Cold water, however, applied to the part is very liable to cause its falling upon the heart, and thus often ending with fatal results. Salves, ointments, etc., are useless. HUMPHREYS' WITCH HAZEL is a most valuable application for the inflamed and swelled parts, and may be applied according to directions on each bottle. ARNICA is often so, but I think not so generally useful as the Extract.

Should there be, during the course of the disease, pain in the region of the heart, oppression or anxiety, jerking, quick or irregular pulse, or other symptoms indicating a transition of the disease to the heart, the Specific No. THIRTY-TWO is appropriate. Dissolve eight pellets in four large spoonfuls of water, and give a spoonful of the solution every two hours, and this may be continued either alone if the disease has been elsewhere subdued, or in alternation with No. ONE, if there is yet fever and heat; or in alternation with No. FIFTEEN if there yet remains merely soreness, lameness, or stiffness of the part. All to be prepared in water, and given at intervals of two hours as above directed.

## CHRONIC RHEUMATISM.

The chief difference between this and the previous form, is the absence of the fever, redness, heat and swelling which characterize the acute form. In old cases, the affected limbs or joints lose their suppleness, and lameness and even permanent curvature or contraction results; and in some cases atrophy or emaciation of the muscles occurs. The causes are the same as in acute rheumatism, and frequent attacks of the latter rarely fail to leave some form of chronic rheumatism as a result.

The symptoms are generally: Lameness, stiffness, or soreness of some particular limb or joint, or of several joints, sometimes manifested on first moving, or on exercise of the affected part, or again principally noticed when quiet. Usually the pains and the lameness are worse on changes of weather, and in rough, damp, windy weather, or on the approach of a storm.

TREATMENT.—Specific No. FIFTEEN, two pellets at a time, and four times per day, before each meal and on going to rest at night, is the appropriate treatment for almost all forms of chronic rheumatism, or for old rheumatic pains in the shoulders, hips, back, chest, side or elsewhere.

If it is associated, as is frequently the case, with some degree of dyspepsia, weak stomach, or constipation, the Specific No. TEN may be taken, two pellets at night, and the No. FIFTEEN as previously directed, before meals.

Rheumatic patients should use largely in their diet, fruit and vegetables, and comparatively less meat. The vegetable acid, or acids of fruit, as obtained in the use of *apples* baked, stewed or even raw. *Lemons* or even oranges, grapes, cherries, etc., are of great use if not invaluable for all rheumatic patients, and should be partaken of freely.

## RHEUMATISM OF THE NECK.

The muscles of the neck sometimes become seriously affected with rheumatic lameness. The head is drawn to one side, or can be turned only slowly and with difficulty, the muscles on that side of the neck are lame and sore when pressed, and there is sometimes fever. It is usually occasioned by exposure to a draught of air, as when sitting near an open window when in perspiration, and is sometimes caused by a sudden jerk of the head.

TREATMENT.—The Specific No. ONE rarely fails to afford relief. Dissolve twelve pellets in six large spoonfuls of water, and of the solution give a spoonful every two hours. In rare cases the No. FIFTEEN may be used, but the No. ONE will usually afford prompt satisfaction. It is needless to say that the neck should be carefully covered and protected from draughts of cold air.

## LUMBAGO—PAIN IN THE LOINS, BACK, NECK, ETC.

This form of rheumatism is confined to the small of the back and the loins, rarely extending upward towards the neck, but more frequently extending down to the hips. There is seldom fever or swelling, or even soreness on pressure, but the pain and lameness is very severe, often almost forbidding motion, or change of posture, as the slightest effort brings on a renewal of the pain.

TREATMENT.—The Specific No. ONE usually affords prompt relief. Dissolve twelve pellets in six large spoonfuls of water, of this give a spoonful every hour, for the first six hours, and then prepare in a similar manner and take at intervals of two hours, until relief is obtained. Should there be any remaining stiffness or lameness, the alternate use of Nos. TEN and FIFTEEN, two pills at a time, and four times per day, will promptly remedy the defect.

## SCIATIC RHEUMATISM.

This form of rheumatism may be attended with some degree of fever, and so may approach the acute form, but in its more common manifestations it is without fever or any considerable degree of heat of the part, and is hence more frequently chronic.

It is characterized by pain, generally sharp, shooting and lancinating, though sometimes more dull and aching in the region of the hip, and frequently extending to the knee or the foot, following the course of the nerve of the affected side. Sometimes it is a dull aching, and may affect only a portion of the limb, or a part of the nervous track mentioned. The pain may be manifested during rest as well as during exercise or motion. It is apt to be tedious, and many persons suffer more or less from it for years in succession.

TREATMENT.—Specific No. FIFTEEN is very generally successful. For the duller and more chronic forms, two pills taken before each meal and on going to rest at night, will be found sufficient. Should there be violent paroxysms of pain, and especially if some heat or fever be associated, give the No. ONE in alternation. Dissolve eight pellets of No. ONE in six large spoonfuls of water, and the same of No. FIFTEEN in another glass, and from these give a spoonful every hour alternately, for six or eight hours, when the interval may be extended to two hours between the doses, and so continue until relief is afforded, when the treatment as for chronic cases may be adopted.

## GOUT—ARTHRITIS.

Gout is generally considered as a dyscrasia or peculiar habit of the body, whereby it is inclined to take a disease of a peculiar form, and when once developed, to render it very intractable or stubborn, and only slightly influenced by the ordinary methods of cure. Its manifestations are similar in form to those of rheumatism, and all the more obstinate cases of this latter disease, or when it is frequently repeated in the same individual, are supposed to be connected with a gouty diathesis or constitution. It is quite liable to be hereditary, but need not be necessarily so, as numerous cases are found where no such transmission is evident, nor is it necessarily the result of an indolent, luxurious mode of life, though its more violent manifestations are commonly due to such a style of living.

The symptoms are usually *extreme pain* in the extremities, often, if not always, commencing at one of the great toes, and thence extending to the foot, ankle, and limb of the affected side. The pain is often extreme, if not insupportable, with extreme sensitiveness of the affected part, which becomes swelled, red, and inflamed. Sometimes it flies from one joint to another, and may even affect the head, stomach, or other part, causing very grave symptoms indeed. When the hands or other small joints have been often attacked, there will be deposits about the joints, which gradually or most frequently harden, causing enlargements, gouty concretions, and rendering the hands or fingers stiff, unwieldy, or even distorted.

THE TREATMENT is the same as for acute or chronic rheumatism, aside from the fact that in gout, or rheumatic gout, the functions of the stomach and kidneys are almost invariably involved, and hence the Specific No. TEN may be profitable, used either as an intercurrent remedy, or in alternation with No. FIFTEEN. Usually No. ONE and No. FIFTEEN for acute attacks, and the latter with No. TEN in alternation for old, chronic cases, will accomplish as much as can be done under domestic management.

## SCROFULA.

SCROFULA is usually considered as a dyscrasia or constitutional vice of the system, manifesting itself most commonly in enlargement and induration of the glands, which may subsequently soften and ulcerate, leaving red or bluish-red discolorations along the course of the opening or eschar. These are often seen along the sides of the neck of old scrofulous subjects. It likewise is supposed to give occasion to enlargement, curvature, or softening of the bones; or more especially the long bones, as of the knee, ankle or hip. These or one of them become sore, tender to pressure, and enlarge at the head, when softening, or ulceration, or necrosis is liable to take place, resulting in the so-called *white swelling* or *hip disease*. Or the dyscrasia may show itself in the form of obstinate eruptions, or even ulcerations of the surface. The swelling of the glands is most frequently manifested about the neck, beneath the ears or jaws, in the form of firm, hard, painless lumps. Scrofula not unfrequently complicates other forms of disease, and renders them obstinate.

Its eradication from the system requires time and perseverance, but may be accomplished by the use of the appropriate remedies. It should be kept in mind that a life-long constitutional taint, requires time as well as proper medicine for its cure; and if eradicated in one or two years, the patient has reason for congratulation. Old school medicine and quackery can do but very little for its cure beyond palliation, while there are numerous cases radically cured by Specific or appropriate Homeopathic medication.

TREATMENT.—For ENLARGED GLANDS about the neck, or in the arm-pits, groins, or other parts of the system, take two pellets four times per day, before meals and on going to rest at night, of the Specific No. TWENTY-THREE, if the swellings are painful, or have suppurated. If they are mere indolent, painless swellings, the medicine taken only morning and at night, will be sufficient.

When these glands become painful or inflamed, and it is thought best to bring them to a head, this will be facilitated and the pain allayed by applications of warm flax-seed, or slippery-elm poultices, which may be renewed from time to time, until the discharge takes place, and they may be continued also afterwards to absorb the discharge, and to promote the healing. To dry up and arrest the discharge, No. TWENTY-TWO, taken two pellets four times per day, will be the proper medicine.

For OLD TUMORS, two pellets morning and night. Though it is not often that they disappear, yet the medicine frequently has the effect of arresting their growth.

For the various forms of SCROFULOUS ERUPTIONS, take two pellets morning and night.

OLD ULCERS require the same treatment, with careful purification of the part, keeping the limb bandaged, if practicable.

## ENLARGED TONSILS.

These often occur in children, called into action from repeated colds or sore throats, or from attacks of tonsilitis, or as the residuum of scarlatina, measles, or similar disease. The tonsils become enlarged, indurated or hard, filling up the pharynx so as to render breathing and deglutition difficult, and the voice often thick or indistinct. The breathing at night becomes especially oppressed, the child at times seeming on the point of suffocation.

TREATMENT.—Excision is frequently practiced, but is not to be recommended, unless in those extreme cases when the tonsils have become so large and hard, as to afford little hope of reduction by medicine, or when the inconvenience or suffering from them is so great as not to admit of delay. In the ordinary cases of children, the Specifics Nos. THIRTY-FOUR and THIRTY-FIVE will be sufficient in reasonable time to reduce them, render them comfortable, and ultimately remove them so far as any material obstruction is concerned. To this end give the No. THIRTY-FIVE, two pellets each morning, and the No. THIRTY-FOUR before dinner, supper, and on going to bed. This is appropriate when there is increased swelling from recent cold, or sore throat. Sometimes in old cases we give No. THIRTY-FIVE in the morning, and No. TWENTY-TWO, two pills at a dose.

## WHITE SWELLING AND HIP DISEASE.

These are usually considered as forms of scrofula, developed in the joints and tendonous structures surrounding it. At first there is occasional limping or lameness, coming on and again disappearing, then more permanent soreness, and tenderness on pressure, and pain at or about the joint, and in hip disease often manifesting itself at some distance down along the limb. Gradually the limb becomes drawn up, painful on exercise; there is heat, sometimes soreness and swelling around the joint, and ultimately suppuration and discharge at some point below the affected joint. This discharge may dry up and again reappear at another joint, and so continue for years until the structure of the joint and its usefulness is destroyed.

TREATMENT.—At first and for any occasional lameness or limping, the No. THIRTY-FIVE is appropriate, and may be given two pills at a time, and three times per day. Should there be some soreness or tenderness at or about the joint, or pain, or swelling, or even after suppuration or discharge, the No. TWENTY-TWO is the proper remedy, and may be given two pills in water, and repeated four times per day, or every three hours if there is considerable pain, heat, redness, swelling, or discharge. This is as appropriate for *white swelling* of *the knee*, as for what is termed *hip disease.*

## GENERAL DEBILITY.

It not unfrequently occurs that persons suffer, or are indisposed from what is termed a *general debility* of the system. When there appears to be no particular disease sufficient to account for the debility of the system, the causes are usually found in either an imperfect assimilation of nourishment, and hence the remedy is to be sought in considering this fault, or the condition occurs as the result of some acute disease, from which the vital forces have been prostrated, and the entire organism weakened and enervated so as not to easily rally, even under the influence of good air and food; or it may occur as the consequence of some drain upon the system, such as a diarrhœa, or leucorrhœa, frequent bleeding, or from similar causes, or it may be induced from mental and physical *over-work*, too great a strain upon the mental and nervous system, with insufficient nutrition. The symptoms are varied, but are generally weakness, easily fatigued on exercise, perspiration on effort, or on going to sleep, weak or lame back, vertigo, singing in the ears, and starting on going to sleep, or slight, unrefreshing sleep, or wakefulness and inability to sleep at night from constant thinking. The above are among the more frequent manifestations.

TREATMENT.—The elements of a cure are first to arrest the drain if such there be, which has occasioned the debility, and then by means of proper nourishment—food that is appropriate, nourishing and easily digested—and by proper relaxation, air and exercise, to restore the wasted substance, and recover the wanted strength. If it is the result of severe, acute disease, only good air, proper nourishment, and even the daily use of some good, generous wine together with the medicine, will be the proper restoratives. If it has been wholly or in part the result of over-work, too much thinking and mental worry or anxiety, coupled, as it often is, with hasty meals and insufficient nutrition, then rest or relaxation, a sea voyage, or other means of intelligent recuperation, are often indispensable. If it is the result of some drain or tax upon the system, too great for its resources, or the result of imperfect assimilation of food, then this drain must be arrested, and such food and medication administered as will correct the evil.

In all similar cases, the Specific No. TWENTY-FOUR is the proper remedy, and may be given two pellets at a dose, and four times per day, always before meals, and on going to rest. It is still more indicated if there be imperfect digestion, wanting appetite, or coated tongue, as well as a general languor and debility of the system.

## NERVOUS DEBILITY.

Closely allied to the above named general debility, is another form of weakness which has obtained the name of *nervous debility.* It partakes of some of the characteristics of the former, and chiefly differs in its origin, and in that the debility is prominently manifested on what might be termed the nervous plane of the organism. It is almost invariably the result of some drain upon the vital forces, such as excesses of various kinds: excessive morbid indulgence, involuntary losses of vital fluids, too long or too constant excitement of the sexual system, and more especially when such indulgences are allowed in connection with mental and physical over-work. This condition is often brought on in young persons from the habit of solitary vice, which persisted in from time to time, is inevitably followed by consequences immediate and remote, which are of the most formidable character. It is safe to say that multitudes are every year brought into the most deplorable condition of nervous debility from these most pernicious practices alone. Parents and teachers cannot be too much on their guard in their behalf, and should deal plainly, kindly, and wisely with such erring ones. The more common manifestations of this condition are: Mental depression, loss of vivacity, buoyancy of spirits and energy, dullness of the eye and the glow of the cheek and lips, love of solitude, and shrinking from society; sometimes loathing or disgust of life to such a degree that suicide is threatened, dullness or confusion of the head, defective memory, or difficulty in recalling names or dates when wanted; the sexual organs are debilitated, relaxed, shrunk up, and in extreme cases wasted; erections are deficient, short, powerless, and in most cases there are involuntary discharges at night during dreams, or during the effort at stool, or during urination. Weakness of the back and loins, general prostration and mental depression and gloom, are the almost invariable attendants. Dyspepsia or weakness of digestion, irregular or capricious appetite, oppression of the stomach after meals, and costive bowels, are very frequent adjuncts. These and other similar symptoms form the picture of a brain impoverished by the loss of its phosphates, and hence performing its functions imperfectly, reflecting its weakness upon the physical system.

TREATMENT.—As in the case of general debility, the first elements of a cure must be to allay the injurious excitement of the organs or system primarily involved; to afford the system proper rest or relaxation, if this debility has been coupled with over-work, mental or physical; to arrest as soon as possible the debilitating drain, and by proper nutrition and medication, to restore the entire organism to its wonted strength and vigor. But all kinds of nourishing food are not appropriate, as some articles otherwise unobjectionable, act too decidedly upon the organs involved, and so tend to induce the involuntary discharges. Thus, eggs, oysters, wine, alcoholic stimulants, or ale, or a strong meat diet, all tend to excite, and hence may promote these losses, and when these exist prominently, the above articles should be avoided. But in the opposite condition, where these discharges are rare, absent or wanting, the diet above mentioned becomes appropriate. In general a *milk diet* is the best, in connection with all refreshing and cooling drinks, fruits in their season, and the lighter kinds of young and white meats. Tobacco, tea and coffee are objectionable, and should be avoided, or used with extreme moderation. To those suffering from involuntary nocturnal discharges, a hard bed, cool room, and but light covering at night are indispensable, and above all, the habit of sleeping *always on the side*, and NEVER UPON THE BACK. As to medicines, the Specific No. TWENTY-EIGHT is the remedy, and may be taken two pellets morning and at night. In some extreme or long-standing cases, a portion of the *powder* No TWENTY-EIGHT may be taken each morning, and the pills as above at noon and at night.

## SLEEP AND SLEEPLESSNESS.

The precise number of hours required for the sleep of each individual daily can be subject to no fixed rule. It differs at different periods of life with the habits, occupation and general health and nutrition of each individual. Some temperaments require more sleep than others, women almost always more than men, and children far more than either. The infant may profitably sleep eighteen of the twenty-four hours; young children may well sleep ten or twelve hours at night, and have an additional siesta during the day, and those that perform severe physical or mental labor, cannot well do with less than nine or ten hours daily. Those who are engaged in light physical or mental labor, will frequently find the wants of nature satisfied with only six or seven hours sleep. Some individuals of remarkable mental and physical endurance, in the midst of the greatest peril or excitement, seem to require but two or three hours of sleep in the twenty-four. But these are exceptional cases. Every individual should take so much of rest and sleep as is required for the restitution of his or her body, strength, and recuperation from fatigue. If nature is long or systematically denied this, there will sooner or later come a terrible retribution, often in failing health, or some nervous disorder or disease of the heart. Several eminent literary men have fallen victims to disease of the heart, attributed solely to incessant mental occupation, carried persistently into the hours which should have been given to sleep. The use of tea or coffee best sustains the system and prevents the waste and wear incident to long watching and severe night work; tobacco may to some extent have a similar conservative effect; but none of them, or all, can more than palliate the serious ill effects of long-continued want of sleep.

The night is the best time for sleep, and it is doubtless true that two hours sleep before midnight is worth as much as four hours after that period. The more nearly sleep can be taken to the hours of darkness, and the earlier we can arise after the morning light the better. From eight or nine o'clock at night, to four, five, or six in the morning, according to temperament, avocation and circumstances, are probably the best hours for repose. During the long warm days of summer, a *siesta* of an hour in the early afternoon is for most persons of leisure as enjoyable as it is allowable, and for young children it is indispensable.

## SLEEPLESSNESS—WAKEFULNESS.

It not unfrequently occurs that persons are unduly wakeful; they either do not sleep soundly, or find it difficult to go to sleep, are easily waked after a short sleep, or their sleep is unrefreshing. Sometimes, while there is an earnest longing, or a desire to sleep, there is a thronging of ideas and restless tossing, that wears away a good part of the night without sleep, or after finally falling to sleep, the slumber is but slight, and they arise unrefreshed, with the demands of the system unsatisfied.

Such a condition has always something of disease or undue excitement connected with it. The excessive use of tea or of coffee may produce it. Too intense or long-continued mental excitement, some forms of dyspepsia or gastric derangement, innervation of the system from insufficient nutrition, or a feverish excitement of the system and afflux of blood to the head, or chronic tendency of blood to the head, may have this condition of sleeplessness or undue wakefulness as a result.

TREATMENT.—In general, Specific No. ONE will be sufficient to afford quiet and refreshing sleep, and more especially when it is occasioned by undue excitement or accompanied with throbbing of the vessels or heat of the head. Take two pellets on going to rest, and repeat them every hour until sleep intervenes. If it seems to arise from mere nervousness, without other apparent cause, use No. THREE in the same manner, two pellets every hour, until quiet sleep is induced. If it has been occasioned by too intense or long-continued mental application, and more especially if connected with indigestion or gastric derangement, the No. TEN, two pellets taken three times per day and at night, will be found corrective.

## NIGHTMARE—INCUBUS.

This disagreeable incident of sleep is dependent upon some morbid condition of the circulatory system, and is too well known to require particular description. It is quite common with some persons, and besides being disagreeable, is not wholly unattended with danger. It will often be found that eating of too heavy, rich or indigestible food, or eating heartily late before going to rest, has been the immediate cause of the attack. When persons are subject to such attacks, or when they are of frequent recurrence, the case should receive careful consideration, and all the occasioning causes of the disease, such as late suppers, heavy, indigestible food, or undue mental excitement, should be avoided.

TREATMENT.—Aside from the hygienic observance above mentioned, the use of Specifics No. ONE or No. TEN will be sufficient. No. ONE, two pellets morning and on retiring at night, when the incubus is attended with heat, fever, thirst, throbbing of the arteries, or heat and fullness of the head. No. TEN, two pills three times per day, the last on going to bed, when there are sedentary habits, constipation, indulgence in wine or other stimulants. For chronic cases, No. ONE in the morning, and No. TEN at night, two pills at a dose.

## PARALYSIS—PALSY.

A limb or portion of the body is said to be paralyzed when it is not under the control of the will, or when the will-power is not able to move or control it. The paralysis may be only partial, or it may be complete, and may affect the nerves of motion only, or may extend to those of sensation as well, so that the part has neither sensation nor power of motion. Sometimes the disease affects only a single limb, and at others the entire one side of the body, or again only the lower extremities.

The disease most commonly comes on suddenly, as the result of apoplexy, or after or during the course of some severe, acute disease. But in some, perhaps most cases, it is preceded by symptoms which, though often unnoticed, should excite attention. These are a sensation of numbness or pricking in one of the limbs, or the entire side, readily going to sleep, as it is termed of the part, coldness or undue paleness of the part, or slight convulsive twitching or jerking of the part or limb involved. When such symptoms are frequently repeated without apparent cause, they should excite apprehension. The causes, aside from those mentioned above, are long continued strain upon the nervous system among men of business, exhausting drains upon the system, and a too luxurious or indolent mode of life, or other similar causes of apoplexy.

TREATMENT.—For the premonitory symptoms: Tingling, pricking or numbness, frequent going to sleep of the limb or parts, No. FOURTEEN is appropriate, and may be given, two pills at a time, and repeated before each meal, and on going to rest.

If there is fullness and redness of the face, heaviness of the head, and disposition to sleep, give No. ONE, two pills at a time, in water, every two hours, for ten or twelve hours, and then give No. TEN, prepared in the same manner, in alternation with it at somewhat longer intervals. For old cases No. FOURTEEN may be given each morning, and No. TEN at night, or if the case is more recent and hopeful, No. FOURTEEN may be given, two pills morning and afternoon, and the same of No. TEN at noon and at night.

## NOSE BLEED—NASAL HEMORRHAGE.

Bleeding from the nose may in some cases be not only disagreeable, but even dangerous. When it is but slight, occurring as it often does in children, or plethoric adults, and attended with fullness and heat of the head, to which the bleeding affords relief, it may be considered almost salutary, and need not be interfered with. But when it occurs in the course of low fevers, consumption, or other debilitating disease, or when it is frequently repeated from apparently slight and insufficient causes, or when it is *severe* and *prostrating*, it should demand attention.

TREATMENT.—Sometimes merely extending the arm and hand of the side upon which the bleeding occurs, upwards over the head, will arrest the bleeding. The application of WITCH HAZEL rarely fails, even in the worst cases. Wet a linen or cotton rag with the WITCH HAZEL folded one or more times, and lay over the nose, covering it from the eyebrows down, and keep this wet with the same, and take ten drops in a spoonful of water every fifteen minutes, until relieved. In extreme cases the WITCH HAZEL may be injected into the nostril with a small syringe, or the nostril may be plugged with lint wet with the same.

If the WITCH HAZEL is not at hand, cold water may be applied to the bridge of the nose, and two pellets of Specific No. ONE may be given in a spoonful of water, and repeated as above every quarter or half hour.

When persons, especially children or young girls, are subject to frequent recurrence of nose-bleed, the use of Specific No. ELEVEN, two pellets taken morning and night, will permanently correct the evil.

## SWELLING OR REDNESS OF THE NOSE.

These affections, though often varying in character and sometimes disconnected, may be conveniently grouped together. Swelling and redness of the nose, more particularly of the extremity, is common among persons addicted to the use of ardent spirits, and among luxurious livers. But it occasionally occurs among the temperate and frugal, causing an unsightly redness of the nose, and a swelling, or even thickening of the integument covering the organ, at once disagreeable and unsightly. The affection is apt to become chronic, increasing from year to year, unless removed by proper regimen and medication.

TREATMENT.—Whether the difficulty has been occasioned by the free use of stimulants, or a luxurious mode of life or not, it is plain that this should be corrected, and a plain diet free from exciting or stimulating food, and absence from stimulants be enjoined. The Specific No. THIRTY-FIVE may be taken, two pellets each morning, and the same of No. FOURTEEN at night. This may be continued until the redness and swelling are removed.

## ULCERATION OF THE NOSE.

The nose, especially the internal nostril, becomes occasionally the seat of frequently recurring ulcerations. The lining membrane becomes sore, ulcerated, crusts form from time to time, and become detached with frequent bleeding.

TREATMENT.—No. THIRTY-FIVE and No. FOURTEEN are curative, and may be used, two pellets morning and at night in alternation, as in case of redness and swelling of the nose.

## SWEATING OF THE FEET.

There are some persons who are habitually subject to perspiration of the feet, which is sometimes excessive in quantity, but more commonly rank or offensive. It is not always permanently removed by bathing, though this is of course important, but depends upon a morbid condition of the tissue involved, the sebaceous glands and follicles, and is a proper subject of medical treatment.

It will be removed by the use of the Specific No. TWENTY-TWO, of which two pellets may be taken night and morning, which may be continued at the discretion of the patient. It is sometimes wonderful, how a few doses of the appropriate remedy will remove an inconvenience of years standing.

## DROPSY.

This term is understood to represent a morbid condition of fluid within some cavity or portion of the system. In itself it is less a disease than a result or product of some diseased condition of the organs or tissues involved. As a consequence, a larger portion of fluid is secreted or deposited than is taken up, resulting in an accumulation of fluid or dropsy. The symptoms or manifestations will vary with the condition of the organs involved, the location and quantity of the fluid, and almost invariably it will be found that the functions of the skin and kidneys, the usual emunctories of the body have become impaired, and that a cure will be effected by their increased activity.

## ANASARCA—GENERAL DROPSY.

The usual symptoms are: An œdematous swelling of the surface of the body and limbs, commencing first on the most depending portions of the feet and legs, and then gradually ascending to the abdomen, hands, face, and other portions of the body. The surface is pale and cold, has a doughy feel, and *pits on pressure.* The secretions become scanty, urine scanty, high-colored, skin dry and bowels confined. Added to these may be symptoms arising from the condition of the organs and tissues primarily involved. It may arise from various causes, among which are prominently—disease or defective action of the kidneys, the localization of the poison of scarlatina, disease of the liver or spleen, and the use of various drugs employed in the treatment of INTERMITTENT FEVER, as arsenic, quinine, etc.

TREATMENT.—The use of the Specific No. TWENTY-FIVE will be the appropriate remedy in this form of dropsy, and may be given, according to the urgency of the case, two pills at a time, dissolved in water, and repeated three times per day for slight cases, or every two hours in the more severe ones.

Dropsical patients require a warm, dry, uniform temperature, and an elevated location if obtainable, with mild, easily-digested food, and the bowels in a free if not relaxed condition.

## DROPSY OF THE CHEST—HYDROTHORAX.

This is one of the most difficult and unmanageable forms of this disease, occurring mostly in elderly people, and often connected with disease of the heart, or protracted pleuritic or pulmonary inflammations. The symptoms are: Difficult, anxious, labored respiration, worse when lying down, or inability to recline, the head must be kept elevated, blueness or pallid face and lips, starting up in affright or dropping to sleep with more rapid breathing, as if in danger of suffocation, scanty secretions and gradual swelling of the feet and abdomen.

The TREATMENT is more difficult and the result uncertain. The Specific No. TWENTY-FIVE may be given, two pellets dissolved in water and repeated every three hours. In case of violent paroxysms of oppression, the No. ONE may be given, a like quantity in water, and repeated every hour between the doses of No. TWENTY-FIVE, as an intercurrent remedy, until the paroxysm has subsided.

In case the dropsy of the chest is complicated with disease of the heart, indicated by irregular or labored action of the heart, the Specific No. THIRTY-TWO may be given in alternation with No. TWENTY-FIVE, two pellets every three hours. Diet and regimen as for general dropsy.

## DROPSY OF THE ABDOMEN—ASCITES.

This is manifested by gradual enlargement of the abdomen, sometimes commencing almost imperceptibly and at others with greater rapidity. The swelling usually commences in the vicinity of the stomach, and thence extends over the entire abdomen. There is with the enlargement difficulty of breathing on exercise, sallow complexion, dry skin, scanty secretions, high-colored urine. There is also a feeling of languor and debility, and stiffness when attempting to bend the body. It may arise from peritoneal inflammation, or from enlargement and disease of the liver, or from some constitutional disturbance.

The TREATMENT is the same as for general dropsy, two pellets of No. TWENTY-FIVE, and given at intervals of two or three hours, according to the urgency of the case. Diet and regimen as for general dropsy.

## OVARIAN DROPSY—OVARIAN TUMOR.

We mention this disease here, as it usually first presents itself in the form of ascites or abdominal dropsy; but in this case there is always a tumor or morbid growth from one of the ovaries, generally the left, which, gradually enlarging apparently from just above the pubic bone, more on one side, extends upwards and over the abdomen, at first more hard and firm, and to which the softer fluctuation of the fluid is afterwards associated, for it is only after the weight and volume of the tumor has compromised the abdominal circulation, that the effusion takes place. When this has occurred, the symptoms are not unlike ascites—large tumid abdomen, œdematous extremities, and scanty secretion with often-disturbed menstruation.

TREATMENT.—The No. TWENTY-FIVE may be given as in general dropsy, two pellets dissolved in water, and administered every three hours.

A remarkable cure was made by the use of the WITCH HAZEL, not only of the effusion but of the tumor itself, and should the No. TWENTY-FIVE fail, I should not hesitate to recommend its adoption.

## INTESTINAL WORMS.—ENTOZOËS.

The human system, in common with the entire animal kingdom, is subject to numerous parasites or *entozia.* These have their abode either upon the surface, or along the intestinal track, or within the cavities, or even in the more solid substances or muscles of the body. They are found in all animals and fish, as well as the human species—those in apparent health as well as those that are sick—and the part they play in the economy of nature is confessedly obscure. It is generally conceded that it is only in peculiar or morbid conditions, or under a course of diet and *regimen* unfavorable to health, that they multiply or increase to such an extent as to become of themselves a source of irritation and disease. It is under these conditions that Intestinal Worms become the subject of medical treatment.

The more important varieties of intestinal worms are :

First—The *seat worm* or *thread worm,* usually called *acarus.* This parasite is from a third to half an inch in length, white, slender and very active. They inhabit principally the lower intestine and rectum. They are more common in children than in grown persons, though the latter are by no means exempt from them. It is not known how these worms originate, since they have even been known in infants at birth. But one fact is well ascertained: that children who live mostly on farinaceous food are most subject to them.

Symptoms.—By their constant and active motions they cause a tickling and irritation in the anus, which obliges the child to scratch and rub the part, as a consequence of which we frequently find a catarrhal inflammation of the mucus membrane of the anus or even a mucus discharge from the part, also a swelling of the veins distributed over the locality, and not unfrequently straining or tenesmus.

From the tendency of these seat worms to travel, they sometimes, in the case of females, enter and irritate the vagina, or in males may occupy the folds of the prepuce, in either case causing intolerable itching and irritation, and occasionally inducing the bad habit of masturbation.

Aside from the medical hints given further on, great care should be taken with children in whom they are discovered, or when from the actions of the child their presence may be suspected, to prevent their accumulation and to remove them. Cleanliness, frequent bathing of the parts, injections of cold water, are generally sufficient to remove the parasites and relieve the irritation. Should it be necessary to remove them from the rectum, this may readily and conveniently be done by injecting an ounce of *olive oil*, with which the worms will usually come away in a mass.

Should the child be restless at night or feverish from the irritation occasioned by them, a dose of two pellets of SPECIFIC NO. ONE will be sufficient to subdue it.

For the permanent eradication of these seat worms from the system, give two pellets of SPECIFIC NO. TWO, morning and noon, and the same quantity of SPECIFIC NO. TEN at night, and continue this course until the object is attained.

SECOND—The *Round Worm* (ASCARIS LUMBRICOIDES) is the next species more commonly met with. It is of cylindrical form, pointed at both ends, from six to nine or even twelve inches in length, and of the thickness of a goose quill, thus resembling somewhat the common earth worm. Its body, however, is half transparent, and of a whitish, yellowish or even brownish hue. They are of both sexes, and the females more numerous than the males.

This worm principally inhabits the small intestines, but it is not unfrequently found in the stomach, and from thence sometimes mounts along up the œsophagus into the throat and mouth, or nose. Attacks of violent, incessant, spasmodic cough are often produced by the attempted passage of a worm into the pharynx. Doubtless, other grave disturbances or morbid conditions are produced, from the presence of these vermin in the neighboring parts.

SYMPTOMS.—These worms may exist in considerable numbers without causing any serious disturbance. But in the majority of cases they *occasion gripings in the abdomen, enlarged or hard, prominent abdomen, mucus diarrhœa*, occasional vomiting, irregular or capricious appetite. There are also from time to time sympathetic symptoms, such as *itching of the nose*, or of the *anus* or *genitals, increased flow of saliva, restless sleep*, with frequent *starting* or *grating of the teeth.* Beside the above more decided symptoms indicating the presence of worms, authors have enumerated the following as manifestations of the worm cachexy : Palor and sickly appearance of the countenance, and occasional flushing of the cheeks; bluish circles under the eyes; dilated pupils; headache or vertigo; voracity or irregular appetite; offensive or fetid breath; acrid eructations; occasional nausea or vomiting; foul or coated tongue; tensive fulness of the abdomen, and gnawing or burning in particular parts of the intestines; hard, tumid abdomen; great thirst; discharge of mucus from the bladder, rectum or vagina; slight febrile symptoms, or erratic remitting fever; nocturnal wakefulness, with low spirits and irritability of temper. We occasionally notice an inflammatory redness of the nostrils, with great disposition in children for picking or boring into the nose, and sudden screaming on awaking, or grating of the teeth in sleep, and involuntary flow of saliva during sleep, also at times, and in sensitive subjects, spasmodic or even convulsive attacks.

These symptoms, indicating the presence of worms, are largely influenced by the regimen and diet of the patient, and even by the season of the year and the lunar phases. Such articles of diet as milk, sugar, preserves, candies and pastry, and sometimes pungent salted food, ham, cheese, etc., produce an aggravation. The leucophlegmatic habit appears to favor their production, and the female more than the male sex.

THIRD—The common *Tape Worm* (TÆNIA SOLIUM). It is only rarely met with in this country. It consists of a *head* not larger than a pin's head, in which there are four sucking cups and their armature; *a neck,* which is an inch or more in length, very slender and without joints ; and *the body,* consisting of a long row of flat, ribbon-like segments, each of which is rectangular in shape and constantly increasing in size towards the caudal extremity. These segments have each the male and female organ, and at the caudal extremity the ripe eggs. There may be several hundred of them, each half or three quarters of an inch in length, and the entire animal may measure several yards. From time to time, the lower segments or joints, as they are termed, ripen, and are pushed off, and appear in the evacuations, and these eggs, being taken by another organism (the hog), form in their organism grubs, and by a subsequent metamorphosis become the original *Tœnia* in the human subject. It rarely happens that more than one of these unwelcome guests are found in the human intestines at the same time, yet there are cases on record where two or more have simultaneously existed in the same person. They are usually found in those regions where people are accustomed to eat raw or not well cooked pork.

The symptoms of *Tape Worm* are all equivocal, unless the segments of the worm itself are discovered in the discharges. Some individuals experience not the slightest inconvenience from it. Others complain of severe pain in the stomach, nausea, vomiting, ravenous hunger, even to fainting. The abdomen is sometimes bloated, sometimes contracted. In some cases there is diarrhœa, in others constipation. Among the sympathetic symptoms are : itching of the nose, vertigo or dizziness, getting dark before the eyes, noises in the ears, palpitation of the heart. These symptoms are ameliorated in most cases by the use of certain kinds of food, such as milk, eggs, mild soups and meat not spiced, while they are produced or aggravated by the use of acids or sour things, especially pickles, spiced with vinegar and pepper, smoked herring, horse radish, cranberries, strawberries, etc. Sometimes, after eating these latter substances, segments of the worm are discharged, and the diagnosis thus established.

For the treatment and permanent removal of the Tape Worm the amateur practioner will be able to do but little. Fortunately, these cases are rare in this country, and where the patient is living wisely, and constantly using appropriate Homeopathic medicine for any occasion that may arise, the Tape Worm will not be troublesome. Practitioners use with success *Kousso* or the flowers of the *Brayera Anthelmintica*, an infusion of two drachms in a tumbler full of water, and letting it stand over night, strain off, and, after taking a cup of coffee to prevent nausea, take half the portion and the remainder half an hour later. The parasite is often carried off after a few hours.

General Treatment.—*Fever* is one of the most common and the most urgent symptoms of verminous irritation, and is usually the more violent in proportion as the worms are higher up in the intestinal track. The fever is characterized by its unsteady character, at times becoming quite violent with red face, or one cheek red and the other pale; white or pale lips or around the mouth; quick pulse; heat of the surface and restless tossing and anxiety; startings on going to sleep, indicating a tendency to convulsions, or even convulsive attacks. It will be generally found on inquiry that the attack of fever has been provoked by some grave error in diet, or exposure, or both—commonly the eating of cake, candy, sweet meats, raisins or other pernicious articles of food, has been sufficient to derange the stomach—to which the irritation of the worms was soon added.

*For such an attack of fever*, dissolve at once eight or ten pellets of Specific No. One in as many teaspoonsful of water, of which give a spoonful every hour, until four or five doses have been given; then prepare of Specific No. Two in the same manner, and give of the two, in alternation, at intervals of an hour, until the fever has abated, when the intervals may be prolonged to two or three hours, until a cure is effected.

Should the fever be quite high, *and there be twitchings*, or startings, or great nervous excitement, rendering the danger of convulsions imminent, loose no time in giving a full *enema* of warm water, so as to secure a free movement of the bowels, and even repeat it, if necessary.

After the storm has passed over, and the fever been allayed, a dose of two pellets of Specific No. Ten, given night and morning, will best restore the normal state of the digestion.

For vague, uneasy or colicy pains in the bowels, arising from the presence of worms, the use of the Specific No. Two, giving two pellets four times per day, will be sufficient. Should it have become worse or complicated by the use of indigestible food, the Specific No. Five may be given instead of No. Two, in the same manner.

*For the permanent eradication of worms* from the system the use of Specific No. Two, giving two pellets four times per day, always before meals, and on going to rest, will be sufficient. If, as in many cases, there is imperfect digestion, or some degree of dyspepsia, the end will be more readily obtained by giving the No. Two—two pellets before meals, and a like dose of Specific No. Ten on going to rest at night.

The Diet in children affected with worms is important. They should not be constantly eating, always "having a piece in the hand." Let them have regular meals, and eat at meal time, rarely except at meals, so that the digestive organs may have rest. Give the child plain, wholesome diet, meat once per day, no pastry, pies, cakes, sweetmeats, raisins or candies, or these as rare and seldom as possible. Under such treatment and management the trouble from worms will be very slight indeed.

## CHOLERA INFANTUM.

Few diseases are more destructive among young children than *Cholera Infantum.* It prevails principally in our cities and larger towns during the hot or summer season, and is mostly confined to children under two years of age. It is much more liable to attack those who are reared on the bottle than those that nurse, and far more fatal or destructive among those who are ill fed, or are living in close, ill ventilated or low rooms, and in the close streets, than among those who have better or wider apartments, or better air. Oftentimes removal to free country air and the use of pure, wholesome milk, is sufficient to effect a cure. To those who cannot remove to the country or to the sea side, the riding on our rivers or bays, in a cool, well shaded boat, is a precious resource. Pure, wholesome food and fresh country or sea air, are often indispensable for a cure in advanced cases.

Symptoms.—The disease generally commences in the form of *diarrhœa,* with frequent, thin or watery stools, which are whitish, yellowish or ash grey, sometimes green or greenish, having a very penetrating, peculiar odor, or sometimes a sourish or sweetish, fresh smell. After a few days, and sometimes from the first, nausea and vomiting is associated with the diarrhœa. The stomach becomes very irritable, vomiting everything that is taken, within a short time, so that nothing seems to be retained. The stools become more frequent or profuse, and the emaciation progresses from day to day. There is usually decided thirst, either from the beginning or after a few days, and the child eagerly watches and greedily drinks of the proffered fluid, often only to have it vomited up again, unless given in very small quantities. Unless relieved, the stools increase in frequency, or become only occasional, but are excessive in quantity and offensive ; the uneasiness, thirst and vomiting increase; the emaciation progresses ; wrinkles form about the nates ; the neck becomes thin ; the skin hangs in folds about the arms and legs ; the face is sallow, pale and shrunken, and the features have an old look ; the eyes becomes dull, and the patient sinks into a stupid slumber, or glides into an "*encephaloid*" condition which, after a day or two, closes the scene.

Sometimes the attack is much more sudden, the child from the beginning having vomiting and repeated thin, watery stools, with rapid sinking and collapse of the system. In the first case, the disease may run from three to twelve weeks, until the child is reduced to a skeleton; or in the latter, or more acute attack, the patient may sink in three or four days.

TREATMENT.—In the treatment of this disease the diet and air of the patient are of first importance. Children who nurse have a much better chance than those brought up by hand, and goat's milk is often better that that of cows, especially for very feeble children. Good, healthy, country air, by preference in an elevated region, or at the sea side, and fresh drawn cow's milk are usually the best sources of restoration, and place the system in the best position to be aided by medicine.

At the first indication of DIARRHŒA, or relaxed bowels, give SPECIFIC NO. FOUR—two pellets, which may be given dry in the mouth, and repeated every two hours—and this medicine may be continued through the entire course of the disease, prolonging the intervals between the doses as the patient improves, or even giving it every hour if the stools are as often, or are *very* frequent. When we have diarrhœa remember to avoid all acids, fruits, tea, coffee, eggs, oysters, chicken or veal, or soup made from them, but use milk, thickened, if need be, with flour, or rice water, or farina. If the child nurses let it be confined to the breast as far as possible, recurring to the above only as auxiliaries.

If the stomach has become *irritable*, the child *vomiting* or *nauseated*, throwing up its food or drink from time to time, the SPECIFIC No. SIX is demanded, and should be prepared by dissolving *twelve pellets* in six teaspoonsful of water, in a glass, of which, after well stirring, a spoonful should be given every hour, and this should be continued until the vomiting and nausea are allayed. Should the diarrhœa continue, and the nausea or vomiting only abated, but not be entirely subdued, and more especially if the stools are quite large, thin or watery, then give the two above mentioned Specifics in alternation, at intervals of one or two hours, according to the urgency of the symptoms, giving two pellets of No. FOUR, dry one time, and a spoonful of the solution of No. SIX the next time, and so on in alternation, so long as the condition requires. Care must be taken in this irritable condition of the stomach *not to give the child food or drink too often, or too much at a time.* Give a few spoonsful, or let it nurse a few moments, then after one or two hours give again, for the stomach often retains a few spoonsful when a larger quantity is rejected, thus increasing the irritability.

If the child moans, frets and worries, is sleepless or tossing about, you can interpose occasionally, as an intercurrent remedy, a few pellets of SPECIFIC No. THREE with advantage.

## KEY TO

# HUMPHREYS' HOMEOPATHIC SPECIFICS.

As this book will doubtless be used by many persons who may have a more or less intimate acquaintance with the usual Homeopathic medicines, and may desire to institute a comparison between the two systems of Homeopathic medication; or in cases where a physician has been called to a patient who has been using the Specifics, and who hence desires to know their composition, in order to have a better understanding of the existing symptoms; I present here, in a tabulated form, the simple medicines of which the several Specifics are composed. Premising also, that these Specifics are all COMBINATIONS, according to the intimation given on pages twenty-eight and twenty-nine, (28 and 29) of the introduction, and generally used in what are termed the middle or lower potencies, or from the third to the sixth attenuation. And I may remark, that the adept in our art, will not fail to recognize the Homeopathic relation of all the medicines named in the several Specifics, to the disease or affection, or to that assemblage of symptoms, which the Specific is designed to cure. And I also promise myself, should health and opportunity permit, at no distant date, to offer the profession "What I know of Specifics," so that nothing of my experience or knowledge in all this behalf, shall be withheld from our common humanity.

No. 1 Cures — **FEVERS, CONGESTIONS,** — Acon. Bell. Bry.

INFLAMMATIONS, HEAT, PAIN.

This Specific is used in all diseases where there is *hot skin, quick pulse,* tossing, restlessness, *extreme pain* or throbbing. For INFLAMMATORY FEVER, with *full, quick pulse, hot skin,* red face, thirst and restlessness.—GASTRIC or BILIOUS FEVER, with quick, full pulse, hot skin, white or yellow coated tongue, bad taste, thirst, nausea, vomiting of mucus bitter or yellow matter, constipation, restlessness, and even delirium.— SCARLET FEVER, with nausea, vomiting, rapid pulse, *sore throat,* hot, red, or mottled skin, scanty urine.— RHEUMATIC FEVER, with full, quick pulse, hot skin, restless sleep, soreness of the limbs, *red, hot, shining, swelling* of the affected part, and scanty, red urine, either alone, or in alternation with No. FIFTEEN.— Violent beating Headaches. — Congestion or rush of blood to the head.— Threatened apoplexy.— Startings on going to sleep.— SLEEPLESSNESS when there is fullness, throbbing, or heat of the head.— INFLAMMATION of the BRAIN, or its coverings.— *Hydrocephalus.* — Violent Ophthalmy.— *Toothache* with throbbing or beating pain, alone, or in alternation with No. EIGHT.—QUINSY or SORE THROAT, in alternation with No. THIRTY-FOUR.— CROUP of the *Inflammatory* or *spasmodic form,* alone, or in alternation with No. THIRTEEN. — CONGESTION of BLOOD to the CHEST. — SEVERE COUGHS, with *hoarseness* and *rough sensation,* fever, or sharp pains in chest or sides. — INFLAMMATION of the LUNGS, with hot skin, quick pulse, oppressed or difficult breathing, heaviness, distress, or sharp pains in the chest, cough, with expectoration of scanty, blood-stained or bloody mucus, alone at first, then with No. SEVEN.—PLEURISY with high fever, quick pulse, intercepted respiration, and *sharp, stinging pain* in the side.— INFLAMMATION of the LIVER, with No. TEN. — INFLAMMATION of the BOWELS, or of the peritoneum.—INFLAMMATION of the KIDNEYS or of the BLADDER, in alternation with No. THIRTY.

## No. 2 CURES } VERMINOUS AFFECTIONS, { CINA. IGNAT. SILIC.

WORM FEVER, WORM COLIC, VORACIOUS APPETITE.

It is used for all conditions supposed to arise from the presence of worms or from a *Verminous Diathesis.* Among these are: Pale face, white lips, enlarged abdomen, with small legs and arms, capricious or voracious appetite, itching of the nose, itching at the anus, too frequent urination, *wetting the bed,* offensive breath, frequent accumulation of water in the mouth. — Versatile fever from the presence of Worms. — TWITCHING of the *face* or *limbs,* or VIOLENT GENERAL CON-

VULSIONS, with holding back of the head, rigid limbs, twitching of the face, etc.—*Hydrocephalic symptoms*, dilated pupils, squinting, etc.—ITCHING of the *anus*.—Seat worms.—Long, round worms.

## No. 3 CURES } DISEASES OF INFANTS. { CHAM. CALC. C. JALAPA.

COLIC, CRYING, WAKEFULNESS, AFFECTIONS INCIDENT TO TEETHING.

It is especially adapted to all diseases of *Infants* and *Young Children*.—COLIC of INFANTS.—CRYING without apparent cause.—SLEEPLESSNESS by day or night, evidently the result of excitement, pain, or unsatisfied desire.—IRRITATION of TEETHING, fretting, worrying, with heated gums and congestion to the head.—*Rash* of Infants.—*Eruption* or *Scurf* on the scalp of infants.—Enlarged and hard abdomen of young children.—SORENESS or EXCORIATION of children.—DIARRHŒA of Infants, or quite young children.—*Twitching* of the *limbs* on going to sleep.—*Convulsions* of Infants.—*Slow growth, slowness* in *learning* to *walk*, tardy closing of the fontanel, and deficient muscular vigor.—Tardy appearance of teeth, or irregularity in the coming of teeth.—SLEEPLESSNESS in ADULTS from overwork, or nervous excitability.—After-pains in lying-in women.

No. 4 CURES | DIARRHŒA. | IPECAC. CHINA. CALC. C.

## DIARRHŒA.

No. 4 CURES — IPECAC. CHINA. CALC. C.

SUMMER COMPLAINT, CHOLERA INFANTUM.

It is peculiarly appropriate to diarrhœa of summer, or the hot season, with *loose, yellow, greenish, mixed or chopped-up,* or even watery stools, with colic or pain.—DIARRHŒA of feeble, emaciated children, attended with nausea, colic, and debility. CHOLERA INFANTUM, in alternation with No. SIX, if there is constant nausea, frequent vomiting, profuse watery, or scanty stools. — DIARRHŒA of children or adults, from indigestion, overloading the stomach, or fat, heavy indigestible food. — DIARRHŒA from the use of fruit, or from change of water or of diet in traveling. — CHRONIC DIARRHŒA, either alone, or in alternation with No. FIVE. — *Dysenteric Diarrhœa,* or *painful Diarrhœa* with mixed stools, streaked with blood. — *Indigestion,* with softness of the stomach, or tendency to diarrhœa.

## DYSENTERY.

No. 5 CURES — COLOC. COLCH. MERC. CORR.

COLIC, TENESMUS, BILIOUS COLIC.

Especially appropriate for COLIC in its varied forms. — FLATULENT COLIC, INFLAMMATORY COLIC, with writhing pain, and tenderness, soreness, extreme sensibility to pressure, or even the weight of the bed-clothes.—Gastric or INTESTINAL COLIC from indigestible substances, alone, or in alternation with No. TEN.—*Bilious Colic*, in alternation with No. TEN.—Specific for FALL DYSENTERY, with colic, tenesmus, bloody, slimy, greenish, mixed, scanty stools, with constant tormena and straining.—*Painful Diarrhœa.*—*Chronic Diarrhœa*, sometimes in alternation with No. FOUR.

No. 6 CURES } CHOLERA-MORBUS. { VERAT. A. ARSEN. CUPR.

CHOLERA, NAUSEA, VOMITING, PROSTRATION.

Promptly curative for CHOLERA MORBUS, with nausea, vomiting, coldness, and even cramps.—As preventive of Asiatic Cholera.—For CHOLERA with coldness, blue surface vomiting, sudden, profuse, thin, or rice-water stools, cramps, and oppressed respiration.—Nausea, or Nausea and Vomiting.—Morning sickness of expectant Women.—Great prostration with coldness.—Asthmatic, oppressed, or difficult respiration.

No. 7 CURES } COUGHS AND COLDS. { BRYON. PHOS. CAUST.

BRONCHITIS, INFLUENZA, SORE THROAT.

It is especially appropriate and curative for all BRONCHIAL and PULMONARY Irritations, and even Inflammations. — HOARSENESS, so as to speak only in whispers, and even entire loss of voice. — Rough, scraping sensation in the throat and pharynx. — Soreness and sense of excoriation in the chest. — COUGH from tickling in the throat. — COUGH from irritation in the bronchia or lungs. — COUGH, with severe stinging pain in the chest or side, expectoration of blood-stained or bloody mucus. — PNEUMONIA, with oppressed breathing, pain in the chest or side, cough and bloody expectoration, either alone or in alternation with No. ONE. — PLEURITIS, with sharp, stinging pain in the side, intercepted respiration and high fever, in alternation with No. ONE. — *Sharp, stinging pains* in the side or chest. — LARYNGITIS, with roughness and scraping in the throat, hoarseness, dry or loose *cough*, and irritation of the throat and bronchia, alone, or in alternation with No. THIRTEEN. — BRONCHITIS, acute or chronic, with dry, irritating cough, hoarseness, or sense of roughness, soreness, or pain in the chest, or even with emaciation and hectic fever towards evening, sometimes in alternation with No. ONE. — INCIPIENT PULMONARY CONSUMPTION, with emaciation, suspicious cough, scanty or frothy expectoration, pain in the chest or side, debility, cold hands in the morning, and slight fever towards evening, or even with perspiration at night, alone, or in alternation with No. THIRTY-FIVE. —

No. 8. Cures } **NEURALGIA.** { Mezer. Plant. m. Bell.

TOOTHACHE, FACEACHE, NERVOUS PAINS.

Especially curative for all NERVOUS PAINS, pains along the course of a nerve, or occupying a limited space, *sharp, stabbing, twinging,* or *shooting,* or with pauses or exacerbations, with extreme nervousness, at times driving one almost to distraction, and without the redness, swelling and heat of inflammation. — TOOTHACHE in partially decayed, or even sound teeth, darting, aching, gnawing, or rending pains, either in the affected tooth, or along the roots of the teeth, or extending to the jaw or face. — TOOTHACHE in OLD DECAYED teeth. — Toothache in sound teeth. — Too rapid decay of the teeth. — PRESOPALGIA or pain in the face, teeth, and jaw, even at times extending to the neck and shoulders. — OLD, LONG-STANDING, inveterate neuralgias, in alternation with No. THIRTY-FIVE. — *Nervous pains,* causing *sleeplessness* at night. — Swelling of the face after toothache.—

No. 9 Cures } **HEADACHES.** { Apis. m. Iris. v. Nux. v.

VERTIGO, SICK HEADACHES, CONGESTION TO THE HEAD.

Appropriate for various forms of *headache,* or of *vertigo,* and for what is termed *rush* of *blood* to the *head.*—Vertigo or swimming of the head, on rising, while walking, or on turning.— Vertigo while lying down.—Constant swimming in the head as if intoxicated.—*Rush* of *blood* to the head, with hot, red face, fullness and heat of the head, sometimes in alternation with No. ONE or No. THIRTY-FIVE.—Chronic fullness of blood in the head.—HEADACHE with beating, throbbing and fullness of the head, red or pale face.—HEADACHE, as if a nail were driven into the head.—HEADACHE, *nausea, vomiting, trembling* and desire to lie down.—*Dull*, heavy, drowsy, stupid headache.— HABITUAL HEADACHES, recurring every few days, brought on by excitement, fatigue or indigestion, attended with *nausea, vomiting, trembling* and prostration, often in alternation with No. TEN.—

No. **10** CURES } **DYSPEPSIA.** { NUX.V. CHIN. SULPH.

DERANGED STOMACH, CONSTIPATION, BILIOUS COMPLAINTS.

Especially curative for GASTRIC DERANGEMENT, or what is often called BILIOUSNESS.—With bad taste in the mouth, coated tongue, offensive breath, want of appetite, constipated bowels, dull, heavy, stupid feeling.—*Evil effects* of a *debauch*, drinking, over-work, or long watching.—Weak, tremulous, debilitated feeling.— HEADACHE from deranged stomach, indigestion, or constipation.—*Vertigo* or *dizziness* of the head, with deranged stomach or constipation.—HEARTBURN.—WATER-BRASH, or *rising* of *water* or *food* to the *mouth*.—DYSPEPSIA, or CHRONIC INDIGESTION, with coated tongue, bad taste in the mouth, offensive breath, rising of water or food in the mouth, belching of wind, spitting up of food or mucus, sensation after eating as of a stone or load in the stomach, fullness or distention of the stomach, slow, torpid, or constipated bowels.—Tenderness of the pit of the stomach when touched.—Light clothes are insupportable.—GASTERALGY, with severe cramp like pain and distress at the pit of the stomach.—CHRONIC CONSTIPATION, slow, hard, knotty, insufficient and infrequent stools.—TOO LONG and TOO PROFUSE *menses*.—LEUCORRHŒA in women, often in alternation with No. TWELVE.—LUMBAGO, or pains in the back or loins.—Bearing down pains in women.—

## No. **11** CURES. } MENSTRUAL IRREGULARITIES. { APIS. PULSAT. SEPIA.

DELAYING, SCANTY, OR PAINFUL MENSES.

Especially adapted to the period of development in Young Women. — DELAYING MENSES in young girls, with chilliness, flushes of heat, pale face, weariness and languor, capricious appetite, etc.— SCANTY MENSES coming only for a short time, then interrupted, or thin, pale color, watery.— SUPPRESSED MENSES, from cold, fright, fatigue or wet feet.—CHLOROSIS or GREEN SICKNESS, with pale face, pale, bloodless lips, easy fatigue, tired feeling, restless nights, capricious or wanting appetite, fetid breath, and *scanty, pale* or *absent menses.—Pale, Leucorrhœaic,* or mucus discharges, instead of the natural menstrual flow. —*Leucorrhœa* instead of the monthly flow, or with scanty menses. — *Ovarian disease,* with enlargement of the abdomen, tenderness in the ovarian region, scanty urine, and irregular menses.— Toothache of pregnant women. — too long or too severe after-pains.—

## No. 12 CURES } LEUCORRHŒA OR WHITES. { CARBO. AN. NUX. V. BELLAD.

TOO PROFUSE MENSES AND PROLAPSUS UTERI.

Especially curative for LEUCORRHŒA or WHITES, *thick, yellowish, cream-like* or brownish discharge, worse before and after the menses, *mild* or excoriating, attended with weakness and debility.— Bearing down pains, sensation as if everything would be pressed out.— PROLAPSUS UTERI.— TOO PROFUSE MENSES.— TOO FREQUENT MENSES.— TOO LONG CONTINUED MENSES, inducing weakness and prostration, sometimes in alternation with No. TEN, or No. TWENTY-FOUR.—Ulceration of the womb.—

## No. 13 Cures } CROUP. { Acon. Spong. T. Kali. B. C.

HOARSE COUGH, OPPRESSED RESPIRATION.

Especially suitable for all diseases or morbid conditions of the Larynx and Trachea.—COUGH hoarse, barking, or with constant inclination to cough, and pain, soreness, or irritation in the throat or larynx.—HOARSE, CROUPY COUGH in children.—COUGH with whispering or hoarse voice, emaciation, soreness of the throat or larynx. —CHRONIC LARYNGITIS, with hoarse or whispering unequal voice, frequent cough, with scanty expectoration, yellow, frothy, or sometimes blood-stained, sense of soreness, scraping, and roughness, as if the larynx was excoriated, emaciation and evening fever.—CROUP, with *hoarse, barking cough, high fever,* and difficult, oppressed, or stridulous breathing.—Spasmodic oppression of the chest, compare No. TWENTY-ONE.—

## No. 14 Cures } ERUPTIONS OF THE SKIN. { Rhus. Tox. Apis. M. Sulph.

ERYSIPELAS, TETTERS, SALT RHEUM, SCALD-HEAD.

Curative for all ACUTE, and even *Chronic Eruptions* of the skin, especially ERYSIPELAS, red swelling, itching or burning, inflamed surface, or with eruption of blisters or vesicles, with high fever and quick pulse, or with deep red swelling and prostration, sometimes in alternation with

No. ONE. — *Nettle Rash,* with large, red or white, raised, itching, wheats or blotches, like mosquito bites, with itching and burning.— ACNE or pimples on the forehead and face of young people. — SALT-RHEUM with chapped, rough, scaly hands, or other parts, often sore or bleeding. — CRUSTA LACTA, or milk crusts in children, with eruption of reddish vesicles, which disclose, forming yellow, and sometimes thick, brownish crusts on the face, forehead, or cheeks. — Old, obstinate eruptions of the legs or body. — Red itching, *eruption in the hairy part of the face,* whiskers and beard often forming thickish crusts. — *Barbers' Itch.* —SCALD HEAD, with eruption of moist vesicles upon the hairy scalp, which, discharging yellow matter, form thick crusts, excoriating the surface, and denuding the hair. — Thick, dark, unclear complexion. — *Old ulcers* on the legs, unsightly, with bluish border, and lardaceous bottom, or with erysipelatous redness around them — consult also No. TWENTY-TWO and No. TWENTY-THREE. — Crusty or scaly eruption coming out in patches, with bran-like scurf, or forming crusts. —

No. **15** CURES } RHEUMATISM. { BRYON. TART. E. ACON.

## RHEUMATISM.

PAIN, LAMENESS, SORENESS.

Especially curative for all forms of *Rheumatism* or vague *Rheumatic pains.* — also for some forms of *Neuralgia* or Nervous pains.—ACUTE RHEUMATISM, with lameness, stiffness, red and hot, or pale swelling of the affected part, intolerable pain on moving, with fever and scanty secretions.—LUMBAGO, with pain and lameness across the loins or back, worse when attempting to walk, and sometimes forbidding an erect posture in walking.—Dull, heavy pains in the loins or back, night and day.—*Pain in the side* or chest, along the intercostal muscles, worse on moving, or by pressing along the affected part.—Pain in the shoulder, extending downwards even to the elbow or hand.—Painful lameness and stiffness of the *nape* or *side* of the neck.—SCIATIC RHEUMATISM with acute pain in the hip, at times even extending to the thigh, leg or foot, of the affected side.—CHRONIC RHEUMATISM with lameness, stiffness, pain, and even curvature of the affected part, principally involving the joints and tendons.—OLD, GOUTY, or RHEUMATIC *enlargements* of the joints, with occasional paroxysms of pain, swelling and tenderness.—Chronic stiffness of the joints.—Lameness of the joints.—Soreness of the integuments as if bruised.—

No. **16** Cures } **FEVER AND AGUE.** { IPECAC. NUX. V CANCH.

INTERMITTENT FEVER, DUMB AGUE, OLD AGUE.

Promptly curative for INTERMITTENT and CLIMATE FEVERS.—*Prevention of intermittent fevers* by persons residing in malarious districts. — BILIOUS SYMPTOMS with coated tongue, offensive breath, bad or bitter taste, no appetite, dullness, easy fatigue, chilliness and constipation, often the forming stage of intermittent Fevers. — FEVER and AGUE with cold chills, with thirst, backache, and pain in the limbs, heat, with thirst, headache, even delirium, followed by perspiration. —FEVER and AGUE, chills, with blue nails, chattering teeth, thirst, pain in back or limbs, heat with headache, sleeplessness, and followed by long-lasting perspiration. — *Fever and Ague, with chills returning every day.* — FEVER and AGUE with chills returning every SECOND day. — Old, partly suppressed agues, with chills returning irregularly, but with constant weak digestion, muscular debility, frequent bloating, bad taste, impaired appetite, irregular bowels, scanty, red urine, and general prostration of the system. — OLD AGUES maltreated by quinine, arsenic, cholagogue, or other nostrums. — Bloating, with enlargement and hardness of the spleen, (ague cake,) in consequence of the ague. — Bloating of the abdomen, and even the entire body from the abuse of quinine. —Has been used efficiently in low forms of fever, approaching Typhus, or Typhoid.—

No. 17 Cures } PILES OR HEMORRHOIDS. { Hamam v. Nux. vom. Sulphur.

External or Internal, Blind or Bleeding.

Especially curative of all engorgements of the venous circulation, and morbid conditions growing out of them.

Piles with sensation as if a stick or hard substance were in the rectum. — Piles with large blue or red tumors which come down at every stool, are returned with difficulty and occasionally bleed, affording temporary relief. — *Large, red* or *bluish* tumors situated at the edge of the anus, intensely sore and painful to pressure. — Bleeding Piles, which bleed at almost every stool, and often at other times, attended with weakness, debility, and broken-back like sensation. — Piles with *prolapsus* of the *rectum* at every stool. — Mucus piles. — *Itching of the anus,* with occasional discharge of mucus. — Internal Piles with painful soreness or lameness in the sacral region, painful, narrow and at times bloody stools.— *Hemorrhoidal colic.*— Constipation *with piles.*—

No. 18 Cures } OPHTHALMY. { Apis. Euphras. Calc. c.

Inflamed Eyes or Eyelids, Weak Sight.

Especially adapted to all morbid conditions of the organs of sight.—*Premature weakness* of *sight,* or in consequence of over-taxing of the eyes in reading, or fine work, or when the system was weak. — Threatened amaurosis. — *Easy fatigue* of the eyes from reading or similar effect. — Intolerance of light. — ACUTE INFLAMMATION OF THE EYES with injected vessels of the conjunctiva, intolerance of light, flow of hot, scalding tears. — OLD OPHTHALMIAS with injection, and even ulceration of the conjunctiva, cornea, cloudy opacity of the cornea, dimness of sight, redness of the lids, and frequent agglutination. — INFLAMMATION, REDNESS, SWELLING or THICKENING of the eyelids. — INFLAMMATION and THICKENING of the margin of the eyelids, denuding the eyelashes. — STYES on the eyelids — Small, painless tumors in the eyelids. — Profuse flow of tears, overflowing the eyelids when in the open air, or exposed to the wind. —

No. **19** CURES } CATARRH. { AURUM. MUR. NITRIC ACID. PULSAT.

ACUTE OR CHRONIC INFLUENZA.

Chiefly adapted to the affections of the mucus membranes, and to the periosteal covering of the bones of the nasal passages. INFLUENZA, with sneezing, flow of hot mucus from the nose and eyes, cough with sore throat, and hoarse, rough, scraping sensation in the bronchia or chest, feverishness and prostration. — CATARRH, with profuse discharge of thick, yellow, or sometimes bloody mucus, obstructed nose, deficient, or sometimes even entire loss of smell. — CATARRH, with impaired sense of taste and hearing. —CATARRH, with occasional discharge of thick plugs of mucus from the nose or throat. — CATARRH, with soreness of the nostrils, crusts or scabs forming in them, with occasional bleeding. — OLD OZENAS, with *sore nostril*, yellow or brownish, thick, OFFENSIVE DISCHARGE, with offensive breath, loss of smell or even of taste, obstructed nose, and sometimes nasal voice. — OFFENSIVE BREATH, with catarrh. — COUGH, with profuse discharge from the nose, and copious expectoration. — LOOSE CATARRHAL cough in children. — OLD SYPHILITIC AFFECTIONS of the nasal bones and throat, with soreness, and copious, brownish or yellowish, offensive discharge.—

## No. 20 CURES HOOPING COUGH. SPASMODIC AND CONVULSIVE COUGHS.

DROSERA. IPECAC. BELLAD. CUPR. M.

Especially curative for irritating and spasmodic coughs.—*Spasmodic cough* coming on in frequent paroxysms, from tickling, or a suffocative sensation in the larynx or throat.—DRY, SPASMODIC cough, with inclination to vomit. — VOMITING of *food during the cough*, and afterwards. — Feeling as of crawling, or of down or feathers in the throat, causing one to cough.—HOOPING COUGH, with frequently returning paroxysms, consisting or a succession of shocks, followed by a deep inhalation or *whoop,* loss of breath, with blueish face, vomiting, raising of mucus, and sometimes convulsive stiffening of the limbs, or holding back of the head. — *Convulsions with the cough.*—*Old, spasmodic coughs,* which seem to take the breath away.— *Cough, with bleeding* from the *nose,* or with expectoration streaked with blood.— *Suffocative fits* during the cough.

No. **21** CURES } **ASTHMA** { LACH. ARSEN. IPECAC.

DIFFICULT RESPIRATION, COUGH AND EXPECTORATION.

Curative for *oppressed, difficult labored* respiration — sensation of heaviness, fullness and weight in the chest. — ATTACKS OF ASTHMA, with labored, difficult, sighing respiration, *cough,* at first dry, irritating, with scanty and gradually with more copious expectoration with relief. — HUMID ASTHMA, with copious expectoration. — Labored, difficult, or oppressed respiration, with throbbing or palpitation of the heart. — *Palpitation of the Heart* with oppression of the chest. — *Cough,* with oppression of the chest. — DRY, IRRITATING COUGH, as if from down or feathers in the throat. — OLD, CHRONIC ASTHMA, with frequently recurring attacks, excited by exposure, over-effort, or mental emotions.

## No. 22 CURES } DISCHARGES FROM THE EAR. { HEPAR. S. PULSAT. SILIC.

EARACHE, NOISES IN THE HEAD, DEAFNESS.

Especially applicable for all affections of the *organs of hearing,* likewise for many morbid conditions and diseases of the *osseous system,* and of *mucus surfaces.* — EARACHE.—INFLAMMATION OF THE INTERNAL EAR, with redness, swelling, extreme sensitiveness of the part, and pain involving the entire side of the head. — Noises, humming, roaring, buzzing or chirping in the ear. — *Hardness of hearing,* with noises in the head. — DISCHARGE FROM THE EAR, as the result of Scarlet Fever, Measles, or from frequent inflammations.— OLD OFFENSIVE DISCHARGES from the ear, with hardness of hearing. — ENLARGEMENT OF THE GLANDS of the neck in children or scrofulous persons. — SCROFULOUS ULCERS of the neck, or old ulcers of the legs of scrofulous subjects. — Intractable ulcers or sores, slow to heal. — *Caries* or *necrosis* of the *bones.* — WETTING THE BED in *scrofulous children.* —

## No. 23 CURES } SCROFULOUS AFFECTIONS. { BARYT. C. LACH. SILIC.

ENLARGED GLANDS, TONSILS, OLD ULCERS.

Suitable and curative for a variety of scrofulous developments, such as : ENLARGEMENT OF THE

TONSILS, filling up the passage and embarassing the respiration and even the deglutition.— SCROFULOUS ENLARGEMENTS of the glands beneath the jaw or ear and upon the neck. — ENLARGEMENT of the *glands beneath* the ARM-PIT, sometimes with inflammation, pain and suppuration. — *Firm, hard enlargement* of the glands like knots about the neck. — *Cold swellings, tumors.* — Tendency to obesity. — Offensive breath of young persons. — *Offensive perspiration* of the *feet.* — *Boils.* — CARBUNCLES, with large, hard, purple swelling, ichorous discharge, with anguish and general prostration. — WHITLOW or FELON. — INFLAMMATION and *ulceration* at the *root* of the *nail,* with severe throbbing pain, with suppuration. — *Old, scaly eruption* on the legs of scrofulous subjects. —

No. **24** CURES } GENERAL DEBILITY. { FERRUM. CHINA. NUX. V.

PHYSICAL AND NERVOUS WEAKNESS.

Curative for DEBILITY in consequence of *severe, acute diseases,* or in consequence of *debilitating discharges,* or *loss* of *blood,* or in consequence of *mental excitement* and *over-work.* — *General tremulous feeling.* — *Feeling* of *weakness* and instability on walking. — *Easily excited,* or made nervous while at work. — Perspiration on going to sleep. — *General prostration,* with feeble digestion, coated tongue, bad taste and deficient appetite.—*Lassitude, tired, weary feeling on* waking in the morning, as if one had not slept enough.—Pale, bloodless lips, and pale face.—Constipated habit.—Ascarides or pin-worms, with itching of the anus. —Compare No. TWENTY-EIGHT.

No. **25** CURES } DROPSY. { APIS. BRYON. ARSEN.

## DROPSY.

FLUID ACCUMULATIONS WITH SCANTY SECRETIONS.

Appropriate for *anasarca*, or *general dropsy*, or with doughy or easily pitting, swelling of the body and limbs, especially the more depending portions.—*Dropsical swelling* of the legs and feet, which pit on pressure.—DROPSY OF THE CHEST, with turns of labored, difficult breathing, inability to lie down, swelling of the feet and legs, or depending portions, and scanty secretion of urine.—DROPSY from BRIGHT'S DISEASE of the KIDNEYS, either fugitive swelling in various parts of the body or face, or permanent, doughy swelling of the feet and legs, with scanty, thick, pale, sedimentitious, or sudsy albuminous urine.—Hydrocephalus of children.—ASCITES or *abdominal dropsy*, with immense distention, œdematous feet and legs, and scanty secretion of urine.—Ovarian dropsy.—Suppressed or scanty secretion of urine.—Copious, pale, albuminous urine.—

No. **26** CURES — SEA SICKNESS. — PETROL. NUX. V. COCC.

VERTIGO, NAUSEA, VOMITING.

Curative for: *Swimming* of the *head,* or vertigo, qualmishness, nausea, vomiting with sinking sensation, prostration and distress. — SEA SICKNESS, with constant *nausea, vomiting,* and utter *prostration.* — NAUSEA, *and even vomiting, from riding* in a *carriage, or on a rail-road.* —MORNING SICKNESS of pregnant women. — *Lumbago, pain,* and *weakness* in the *loins,* which does not permit standing upright. — Paralysis of the lower extremities. — Paralytic weakness of the loins and back. —

No. **27** CURES — KIDNEY DISEASES. — PULSAT. LYCOP. SARSAP.

RENAL CALCULI, GRAVEL, PAINFUL URINATION.

It is found curative for various morbid affections of the kidneys, manifested by: Pain, uneasiness or lameness in the loins or kidney region, thick, muddy, or sedimentitious urine, occasional deposits of sand, gravel, or reddish brick-dust, or white, pus-like matter. — *Renal colic,* with violent pain in the back, extending forward and downward, or involving the entire abdomen, sometimes with retraction of the testicle, and scanty or blood-stained urine. —RENAL CALCULI. —Difficult urination, with slow, interrupted stream. — Too

FREQUENT urination.— Must rise several times in the night to urinate. — ENURESIS of *old people.* — Old disorganizations of the kidneys. —*Strangury,* with urgent desire and discharge of mucus, and white, thick deposit. — Burning while passing the water. —BLOODY URINATION, *discharge* of *urine mixed with blood.* —

## No. 28 CURES. NERVOUS DEBILITY. PHOS. AC. CHINA. AURUM.

### SEMINAL WEAKNESS, DEFICIENT ENERGY.

Specific for all conditions arising from *exhaustion* of the *vital powers, loss of vital fluids, excessive drains,* or over-taxing the system. — CONSEQUENCES of YOUTHFUL VICES, *indiscretions,* or *abuse,* manifested by: Easy forgetfulness, irresolution, shamefacedness, avoidance of society, love of solitude, pale face, depression, gloomy, taciturn mood, loathing of life and great bodily weakness, *repugnance* to *exercise,* or physical or mental effort. — FREQUENT, INVOLUNTARY, SEMINAL *discharges,* with lascivious dreams, followed by increasing prostration. — POLLUTIONS *from relaxed organs.* — *Emission too soon,* too rapid. —WEAKNESS of the SEXUAL ORGANS, which remain flaccid, with deficient erectile power. — *Debility* of the *organs* in consequence of over-indulgence or excesses. — *Mental alienation,* caused by masturbation.

No. 29 Cures } **APTHÆ OR SORE MOUTH.** { Nat. mur. Nux. vom.

**Canker, Ulcerated Lips.**

Curative for the Sore Mouth of *Infants*, consisting of minute red points, which soften, leaving white patches of ulceration, which often extend over large surfaces, attended with soreness, scalding, and burning. — Sensation as if the mouth and tongue had been scalded with hot tea. —Apthæ of adults, or patches of ulceration on the tongue, lips, or inside the cheek, with flow of water, soreness and burning of the affected part. — Sore mouth of nursing women. — Mercurial and Syphilitic sore mouth, almost the entire buccal cavity is raw and sore, as if excoriated, hot, scalding and burning. — Obstinate, Intermitting Fevers, with predominating headache during the paroxysm. — *Ulceration* of the *corners* of the *mouth.* — Sore, ulcerated or chapped lips. — Tetter-like eruption around the mouth. — Tardiness of children in learning to talk, from difficulty in using the tongue. —

No. 30 Cures } **URINARY INCONTINENCE.** { Cann. Canth. Merc.

**Frequent, Painful or Scalding.**

Curative especially for *Inflammatory* or *sub-inflammatory conditions* of the *urinary organs.* —

INFLAMMATION of the KIDNEYS, with fever, pain across the loins, frequent discharge of hot, dark-red, or even bloody urine, attended with burning and pain, which often extends down the inside of the limb.—Constant desire to pass water, and inability to restrain it.—INFLAMMATION of the BLADDER, with pain in front over the pubes, constant desire to pass water, and painful discharge of scanty, high-colored, or even bloody urine.—Fruitless straining, passing only a few drops at a time.—*Urine loaded* with mucus or pus.—INFLAMMATION of the URETHRA (GONORRHŒA) with frequent, scalding, burning urination, and inability to retain it, discharge of thick, yellow matter from the urethra, and swelling of the prepuce.—*Discharge* of THICK, YELLOW, or whitish matter from the urethra, with slight scalding or irritation.—WETTING the BED NIGHTLY, URINARY INCONTINENCE in children, or even older persons, obstinate cases of verminous children may also require No. TWO, or scrofulous subjects may also require the No. TWENTY-TWO.—

No. **31** CURES } PAINFUL MENSES. { PLAT. COCCUL.

HYSTERIA, PRURITIS, SPASMS.

Curative for a variety of forms of *Dysmenorrhœa* or *painful menstruation* and *Hysteria.*—PAINFUL PRESSURE and BEARING DOWN, *before and during the menses,* with extreme sensibility of the parts.—

CRAMPS, or even GENERAL SPASMS at the *commencement* of the *period.* — *Cutting* pains like those of labor before the menses. — VOLUPTUOUS CRAWLING, ITCHING and *irritation* of the *genital organs,* almost driving one to distraction. — *Delaying* or *suppressed menses,* with colic or cramping pains, nausea, spasm of the chest, and cramps or convulsive movements of the limbs. — Laughing, crying, or hysterical movements or cramps, at the commencement of the monthly flow. — Too COPIOUS and LONG-CONTINUED menses, with itching and irritation of the parts. — Too LONG continued menses, with leucorrhœa in the interval. — Too EARLY, and TOO LONG-CONTINUED menses. — *Leucorrhœa* like the *white* of *eggs.* — Discolored, dirty-looking leucorrhœa. —

## No. 32 CURES } CLIMACTERIC INCIDENTS. { LACH. SEPIA. CACTUS.

IRREGULARITIES, FLUSHES, PALPITATIONS.

Indispensable for the irregularities and accidents incident to the climacteric changes of women. — Headache during the menses. — IRREGULAR MENSTRUATION, now too soon and too copious, and then delayed and scanty. — Too COPIOUS MENSES, almost like flooding, continuing several days, and inducing great prostration. — *Delayed* or *failing menses,* with vertigo, fullness and heat of the head, and general heaviness of the body. — FLUSHES of

HEAT suddenly coming over one, with hot, red, or pale face, and then vanishing with a sense of faintness and perspiration. — PALPITATION, BEATING or *violent throbbing* of the *heart,* in connection with irregularities.—Oppression and weight in the chest. — Paralytic heaviness of the chest, as if one could not get the air. — PALPITATION *of the heart.* — IRREGULAR ACTION and tumultuous beating of the heart. — *Painful spasm* through the *chest* and *heart,* with a sinking, death-like sensation. — RHEUMATISM of the HEART. — *Old, chronic palpitations* or *disease* of the *heart.* —

No. **33** CURES } EPILEPSY. { IGNAT. BELLAD. SULPH.

## EPILEPSY.

CRAMPS, SPASMS, CONVULSIONS.

Especially curative for various morbid conditions of the *nervous* and *cerebro-spinal* systems. — *Twitchings* or involuntary movements of single muscles or limbs. — Grimaces of the face, or strange drawing of the features or muscles. — CHOREA ST. VITI, with twitching of the face, arms or limbs; involuntary movements, jerks, unsteady walking, dropping of things, and nervous excitability. — CONVULSIONS of CHILDREN from teething, irritating food, fright or mental excitement, with holding back of the head, rigid and then convulsed arms and limbs, purple face, frothing at the mouth, and unnoticed evacuations. —

*Cramp* of *single limbs.*—*Easy becoming numbed,* or *going to sleep* of the *limbs.*—*Cataleptic stiffness* of the *limbs* or *body.*—EPILEPSY, with cries, falling down, foaming at the mouth, convulsed face and limbs, retracted thumbs, and involuntary evacuations.—*Paralytic numbness* and *insensibility* of *one side.*—

No. **34** CURES } DIPHTHERIA. { PHYTOL. LACHESIS. MERC. PROT.

QUINSY AND ULCERATED SORE THROAT.

Curative for TONSILITIS, with redness, swelling and stinging pain in the tonsils, and soft parts, difficult, painful deglutition, fever and thirst.—Painful, difficult swallowing.—Inability to open the mouth from the swelling, choking sensation in the throat.—QUINSY, with redness, swelling and inflammation of the entire throat and fauces, painful or impeded deglutition, the fluid sometimes returning by the nose, pain in the head, fever and thick coated tongue.—ULCERATED SORE THROAT, with painful or impeded deglutition, offensive breath, and discharge from the throat, heavy coated tongue, swelling of the glands of the neck, and fever prostration.—DIPHTHERITIC SORE THROAT, with high fever, red face, *swelling* of the *glands* of the *neck, unusual prostration* of the system, headache, fever, SWELLING of the TONSILS, UVULA, and SOFT PARTS, *which are cov-*

*ered with dirty patches of ulceration.*—Old chronic, often returning, sore throats. — CHRONIC ENLARGEMENT and *induration* of the *tonsils*, also No. THIRTY-FIVE. –

No. **35** CURES } CHRONIC CONGESTIONS. { BELLAD. CALC. C.

HEADACHES AND ERUPTIONS.

Curative for chronic congestion, heat, fullness and pressure of the head.—Dizziness, Vertigo, and swimming of the head. — HABITUAL HEADACHES. — HEADACHE, with fullness, pressure or pulsation in the forehead, or on one side. — *Violent throbbings* or *stabbings* in the head. — HEADACHE from *study, over-work*, or *mental effort*.— Indisposition or inability to study, or to make any considerable mental effort, in children.— — INFLAMMATION of the EYES from reading or overtaxing the sight. — SCURFY ERUPTION on the heads of infants. — HUMID, SCABBY ERUPTION or tetter on various parts with burning. — Swelling and induration of the glands, sometimes with pain and heat. — Muscular weakness. — DIFFICULTY of CHILDREN IN LEARNING TO WALK. — Retarded *closing* of the fontanel. — Irregular or slow appearance of the teeth. — SLEEPLESSNESS IN CHILDREN, RETARDED SLEEP and RESTLESSNESS in adults, from nervousness and flow of ideas, with lassitude and weariness in the morning, as if one had not slept.—Too EARLY and too LONG continued *menses* in *women.* — Too COPIOUS or *excessive menses.* — *Prolapsus uteri* constant and *bearing down.* — LEUCORRHŒA. — COUGH with *pain in the side.* — COUGH with pain and oppression of the chest, and copious expectoration.—SUSPICIOUS COUGHS in young, delicate, consumptive subjects. — *Constant liability to take cold* from slight exposure.

# INDEX TO FOREGOING KEY

AND THE

# SPECIFICS INDICATED BY THE VARIOUS SYMPTOMS.

# GLOSSARY OF MEDICAL TERMS

## USED IN THIS WORK.

### A.

ABORTUS.—Miscarriage ; abortion.

ACETUM.—Vinegar.

ACNE.—An eruption consisting of small pimples, mostly on the face.

ACNE ROSEA.—A redness of the nose and cheeks; found often in persons much addicted to the use of ardent spirits.

ADENITIS.—Inflammation of the glands.

ADYPSIA.—A lack of thirst.

AGALACTIA.—A defect of milk in childbed.

AGGLUTINATION.—The adhesion of parts to each other.

AGRYPNIA.—Sleeplessness.

ALLOPECIA.— Baldness ; fall of the hair.

AMBLYOPIA.—Dimness of sight.

AMENORRHŒA. — Stoppage of the menstrual discharges.

AMIGDALITIS.—Inflammation of the tonsils.

ANEURISM.—A preternatural tumor, formed by the dilatation of an artery.

ANASARCA.—A species of dropsy between the skin and flesh.

ANGINA.—A sore throat, (difficulty of swallowing.)

ANOREXIA.—A want of appetite, without absolute loathing of food.

ANOSMIA.—Loss of the sense of smelling.

ANTHROPOPHOBIA.—Dread of society.

APHTHÆ.—Frog, sore mouth, a kind of ulcers which spread sometimes, over other parts of the body.

APHONIA.— A suppression of the voice.

ARTHRITIS.—The gout.

ARTHROCACE.—"Ulcer in the cavity of the joint bone."

ASCITES.—General dropsy.

ASCARIDES.—A genus of intestinal worms.

ASTHENIC INFLAMMATION—Passive inflammation.

### B.

BALANITIS.—Inflammation of the glans penis.

BALANOBLENORRHŒA.—Pseudo gonorrhœa.

BLEPHAROPTHALMIA. — Inflammation of the eyelids.

BLEPHAROSPASMA.—Spasm of the eyelids.

BORBORYGMI.—A noise occasioned by wind in the intestines.

BRONCHITIS.—Inflammation of the air-tubes.

BUCCAL HAEMORRHAGE.— Haemorrhage from the mouth.

### C.

CACHEXIA.—A bad habit of body.

CARDITIS.—Inflammation of the heart.

CALCULUS.—Stone, as for instance in the bladder.

CARPHOLOGIA—A delirious picking of the bed-clothes.

CARIES.—Rottenness, mortification of the bones.

CATALEPSY.—A sudden suppression of motion and sensibility.

CEPHALGIA.—Headache.

CERUMEN.—Wax, for instance.

CHLOROSIS.—Literally the green disease; a disease peculiar to young females.

COMA.—An inclination to sleep, a lethargic drowsiness.

COMA VIGIL.—An inclination to sleep, but inability to do so.

CORYZA.—A cold in the head.

COXALGIA.—Pain in the hip-joint.

COXARTHROCACE.—Hip-disease.

CUTIS ANSERINA.—Goose pimples.

CRUSTA LACTEA.—An eruption attacking the face and head of nursing infants.

CYANOSIS.—"The blue disease."

CYNANCHE—Angina, sore throat.

## D.

DECUBITUS.—Soreness, caused by long confinement to one position in bed.

DIABETES.—Urinary flux.

DIATHESIS.—A predisposition to the development of a particular disease.

DIAPHRAGMATIS.—Inflammation of the diaphragm.

DIABETES.—An immoderate discharge of urine.

DIURESIS.—An increased secretion of urine.

DYSCRASY.—A peculiar ill-habit of body or constitution.

DYSECOIA.—Difficulty of hearing.

DYSPHAGIA.—Difficulty of swallowing.

DYSMENORRHŒA.—Difficult or painful menstruation.

DYSPNŒA.—Difficult respiration.

DYSURIA.—A suppression of, or difficulty in voiding urine.

DYPLOPIA.—Double vision.

## E

ECTROPIUM.—An eversion of the eyelids.

ECLAMPSIA.—A scintillation, flashing of light which frequently strikes the eyes of epileptic persons.

ECCHYMOSIS.—A black or blue swelling, either from a bruise, or a spontaneous extravasation of blood.

ECZEMA.—Humid tetter, or moist eruption of the skin.

EMPROSTHOTONOS.—A clonic spasm of several muscles, which keeps the body in a fixed position, bent forwards.

ENTERALGIA.—Pain in the bowels.

ENEURESIS.—Incontinence of urine.

ENCEPHALITIS.—Inflammation of the brain.

ENCYSTED TUMOR.—A fluid tumor enclosed in a sac.

ENTERITIS—Inflammation of the intestines.

EPHELIS.—A sun spot.

EPISTAXIS.—Bleeding from the nose.

EXOSTOSIS.—A morbid enlargement or tumor of a bone.

## F.

FONTANEL.—A space occupied by a cartilaginous membrane in the new-born child, and situated at the union of the angles of the bones of the cranium.

FORMICATION.—A sensation as if ants were running over the skin.

FUNGUS-HÆMATODES.—A bleeding tumor.

FURFURACEOUS TETTERS.—Bran-like tetters.

FURUNCULI.—Boils.

## G.

GALACTORRHŒA.—Flowing of the milk.

GANGRENE.—Mortification.

GASTRALGIA.—Pain in the stomach.

GASTRITIS.—Inflammation of the stomach.

GLANCOMA.—An opacity of the vitreous humane of the eye.

GLOSSITIS.—Inflammation of the tongue.

GLOSSOPLEGIA.—Paralysis of the tongue.

GONITIS.—Inflammation of the knee.

## H.

HÆMATOCELE.—A swelling of the scrotum, proceeding from blood.

HŒMATEMESIS.—Vomiting of blood.

HÆMATURIA.—Voiding of blood with urine.

HÆLOPTYSIS.—Spitting of blood.

HELMINTHIASIS.—A disease by which worms or larvæ are bred under the skin.

HEMERALOPIA.—A defect in the sight, in consequence of which the person sees only during the day, not at night.

HEMIOPIA.—A defect of sight, when the person sees only one-half, not the whole of the object.

HEMIPLEGIA.—A paralytic affection of one side of the body.

HEPATITIS.—Inflammation of the liver.

HERNIA.—A protrusion of the intestines.

HERPES.—A species of eruption.

HIPPOCRATICAL-FACE.—A particular disposition of the features of the face preceding death.

HORRIPILATION.—A sensation of shuddering or creeping.

HORDEOLUM.—A little tumor on the eyelid resembling a barley corn ; Stye.

HYDRARTHRA.—Dropsy of the joints.

HYDROTHORAX.—Water in the chest.

HYDRARGYROSIS.—Mercurial disease.

## I.

ICTERUS.—The jaundice.

ICTHYOSIS.—A species of eruption.

IMPELIGO.—A disease of the skin.

INGUINAL HERNIA.—A rupture of the intestines appearing in the groin.

INTERTRIGO.—An excoriation about the anus, groins, or other parts of the body.

ISCHURIA.—(Spasmodic) retention of urine.

## L.

LARYNGITIS.—Inflammation of the larynx.

LIENTERIA.—Diarrhœa, where the food passes off undigested.

LIPPITUDO.—An exudation of a puriform humor from the margin of the eyelids.

LITHIASIS—A formation of stone or gravel.

LUMBRICI.—Round worms.

## M.

MARASMUS.— Emaciation, M. Seniles, the wasting away of old people.

MEGRIM.—A species of headache on the side of the head.

MELÆNA.—The black vomit.

METRITIS.—Inflammation of the uterus.

MENOCHEDIA.—Too scanty menstruation.

MENOPOSIA.—Critical age of women.

MENOSTASIS.—Stoppage of menses.

METRALGIA.— Spasms in the uterus.

MENTAGRA.—An eruption about the chin.

METRORRHAGIA.—An excessive discharge of blood from the uterus.

MILIARY eruptions.— Eruptions of small vesicles on the skin, resembling millet seed (milium), hence the name.

MORBILLI.—The measles.

MYELITIS.—Inflammation of the spinal marrow.

MYOPIA.—Nearsightedness, purblindness.

## N.

NAEVUS.—A natural mark.

NARCOTISM.—Stupor.

NECROSIS.— Mortification of bone.

NEPHRALGIA.—Pain in the kidney.

NEPHRITIS.— Inflammation of the kidney.

NEURALGIA.—Pain in a nerve.

NODUS.— A tumor proceeding from a bone.

NOSTALGIA.—Home-sickness.

NYCTALOPIA.— Inability to see in the day time.

## O.

OBESITY.—Corpulency.

OCCIPUT.—Back part of the head.

ODONTALGIA.—Toothache.

OEDEMA.—Dropsical bloating of a portion of the surface.

OESOPHAGITIS.—Inflammation of the gullet.

OPHORITIS.— Inflammation of the ovaria.

OPHTHALMIA.—Inflammation of the eye.

OPISTHOTONIS.— Spasms of the muscles by which the body is bent backwards.

ORCHITIS.—Swelling of the testicle.

ORTHOPNŒA--Laborious breathing, which obliges the person to sit erect.

OTALGIA.—Earache.

OTITIS.— Inflammation of the internal ear.

OTORRHŒA.—A discharge from the ear.

OTORRHAGIA.—A running from the ear.

OZÆNA.—A peculiar fœtid discharge from the nose.

## P.

PALPIPATIS Cordis.—Palpitation of the heart.

PANARIS.—See whitlow.

PAROTIS.—A gland (Parotid) beneath the ear.

PAROTITIS—Inflammation of the parotid gland.

PEMPHIGUS.—A fever attended with a successive eruption of vesicles.

PERITONITIS.— Inflammation of the lining membrane of the abdomen.

PETECHIA.—A red spot resembling a flea bite.

PHAGEDEMIC.— An ulceration which spreads rapidly.

PHLEGMATIS. Albadolens.—An affection of the lower limbs of women during or after childbed.

PHOTOPHOBIA.—Intolerance of light.

PHTHISIS PULMONARIS.—Consumption of the lungs.

PHTHISIS FLORIDA.—Rapid consumption of the lungs.

PHTHISIS.—Phlegm consumption.

PHTHISIS.—Consumption of the kidneys.

PITUITA.— Phlegm or viscid mucus.

PLETHORA.—A redundance of blood.

PLEURA.—The lining membrane of the chest.

PLEURITIS OR PLEURISY.—Inflammation of the pleura.

PLEURODYNIA.—Pain in the pleura or side.

PLICA POLONICA.—Matted hair, peculiar to Poland.

PNEUMONIA.— Inflammation of the lungs.

PODAGRA.—Gout.

POLYPHAGIA.— Great desire to eat.

POLYPUS.—A pendiculous tumor with a small neck and without sensibility.

POLYSARCIA.— Troublesome corpulency.

PORRIGO.—A disease of the hairy scalp.

PRESBYOPIA.—Obscure vision.

PROLAPSUS RECTI. A protrusion of the rectum.

PROLAPSUS UTERI.— A falling down of the womb.

PROSOPALGIA.—Pain in the face.

PROSTATITIS.—Inflammation of the prostate gland.

PRURIGO.—A cutaneous disease.

PSEUDOPIA.—False sight.

PSOITIS.— Inflammation of the sheath of the psoac muscles.

PSORA.—See scabies.

PSORIASIS--A species of scabies. See scabies.

PTYALISM.—Salivation.

PTYRIASIS.—Dandruff.

PUERPERAL PERITONITIS.— Inflammation of the lining membrane of the abdomen after child-birth.

PURPURA.—A purple eruption attended with debility.

PYROSIS.—The water-brash.

## R.

RANULA.— A tumor under the tongue caused by the obstruction of the ducts.

RACHITIS.—The rickets.

RAGHADES.—Chaps.

RISUS SARDONICUS.— Sardonic laughter.

RUBEOLA.—The measles.

RUPIA—A flat vesicular eruption.

## S.

SABURES.—Dirt, sordes.

SATURNINE COLIC.— Colic caused by lead.

SCABIES.—The itch.

SCALDHEAD.—See Tenia Capitis.

SCIATICA.—Pain in the sciatic nerve.

SCIRRHUS.—A hard, and almost insensible tumor.

SCORBUTUS.—The scurvy.

SINCIPUT.—The fore part of the head.

SPLENALGIA.—Pain in the spleen.

SPLENITIS.—Inflammation of the spleen.

SPHACELUS.—A mortification of any part.

STEATOMA. — An encysted tumor of a sooty consistence.

STOMACACE.—Similar to scurvy.

STRABISMUS.—Squinting.

STRANGURY.—A difficulty in making water.

STROPHULONS.—An eruption peculiar to infants.

SYNCOPE.—Fainting.

## T.

TABES DORSALIS.—Wasting of the body.

TABES MESENTERICA.—A disease of a set of glands situated in the abdomen.

TÆNIA.—The tape-worm.

TENESMUS.—A continual inclination to go to stool.

TETANUS.—Spasm, with rigidity.

TENIA CAPITIS.—An eruption of small ulcers at the roots of the hair.

TETTER.—See Herpes.

TRACHEITIS.—Inflammation of the trachea.

TRICHIASIS.—A disease in which the eyelashes are turned inwards.

TRAUMATIC CONVULSIONS.—Convulsions caused by a wound.
TRAUMATIC FEVER.—Fever following a wound.
TRISMUS.—Locked jaw.
TYMPANITIS.—An elastic distension of the abdomen.

## U.

URTICARIA.—Nettle rash.

## V.

VARICELLA.—Chicken-pox.
VARICES.—A distention of the
VARIOLA.—Smallpox.
VERTIGO.—Giddiness.
VESICA.—The bladder.

## W.

WHITLOW.—A collction of pus in the fingers.

## Z.

ZONA.—Shingles.

# GENERAL INDEX.

# HUMPHREYS' WITCH-HAZEL;

## THE MARVEL OF HEALING.

### HISTORY AND USES.

THERE are some shrubs or trees that seem marked by nature for extraordinary uses; among these, the WITCH-HAZEL affords a striking example. It is a modest, unpretentious shrub, seldom growing more than six or eight feet in height, with several crooked branching stalks an inch or two in thickness, growing from a common root, having a smooth, spotted bark, and smooth, somewhat thickish, serrated leaves. It is common in most parts of the United States, and found in good soil around springs and running waters, along the margins of streams, or on the high hills overlooking them. Its leaves are put forth late in Spring, and during the late Autumn or Fall, when the American forest is clothed in the thousand gorgeous hues of Indian Summer, and other shrubs and trees drop off the ripened leaves, this shrub, as if to attract attention to its primeval usefulness, amid the year's decay, throws out its mild yellow blossoms, and till late Winter storms, and amid deep snows, cheers the desolation with its flowering petals.

FROM the earliest settlement of our country, somewhat of superstition, and much of popular veneration, has been recorded concerning it. The Indians doubtless used it, and taught the early settlers something of its value. From its branches the "Divining Rod" was made, with which those who practiced the occult art, located wells or underground springs, or water courses, or beds of mineral ore. Others used the shrub in various ways for different forms of disease or illness. Sometimes a tea was made from its bark or root, and given to those afflicted with diarrhea, spitting of blood, or pains in the chest. Often a poultice of the pounded bark was laid upon old sores, hot swellings, or chronic ulcers; while others took simply the tender branches, and denuding them of the rough bark, rubbed these "sticks" over the sores, ulcerations, or burns, and thus healed them. The wide-spread use of the shrub in these many ways, is evidence of its great curative properties. Though doubtless not always curative when used in these crude and bungling ways, yet it was sufficiently often so to sustain its general reputation, and to extend its use and good name among the people.

VARIOUS crude and imperfect attempts were made at divers times to prepare a medicine from the WITCH-HAZEL which should develope and preserve, in a conveneint and concentrated form, its entire curative properties,—which should be accompanied by a history and statement, pointing out the diseases, morbid conditions, and injuries which it would cure,—and which should finally show how the medicine thus prepared should be applied in the most safe, convenient, and advantageous manner. A failure in either of these points, is fatal to the scheme of making the remedy a truly **popular medicine.** One Theron Pond, in a preparation which he called "Pond's Extract," did something in that way. But those crude efforts of mere laymen, unacquainted with the science or art of medicine, never accomplished anything of note. It required the efforts of a scientific and skillful physician, of large observation, extensive research and practical skill, to bring the resources of his knowledge and experience to the solution of this subject. DR. HUMPHREYS gave Pond his best ideas on the subject of its preparation, and for more than twenty years he has made the preparation and curative properties of this shrub the subject of his study, observation and research. He has written nearly everything about it, and has made its development and preparation the object of his especial care, so that no man knows so much about it, or so well how to prepare it, as he.

HUMPHREYS' WITCH-HAZEL contains, in its most active and concentrated form, the **entire curative properties** of the WITCH-HAZEL, sometimes called the *Spotted Alder* or **Hamamelis Virginia.** This medicine is obtained by a process of distillation and subsequent treatment, through which the woody and coloring matter is rejected, and the natural aroma, curative and diffusive properties, are developed and preserved. It forms a clear or slightly milky fluid, with a specific gravity above that of water, having a peculiar aromatic and diffusive taste, and, taken in the mouth, instantly pervades the system. The odor or aroma is peculiar and diffusive and to most persons not at all disagreeable. It is put up in 6 oz., pint, and, quart bottles, having the name "HUMPHREYS' WITCH-HAZEL" upon the labels and blown in the bottles, and is accompanied by the WITCH-HAZEL book of directions. It is free from the dirt, soot, and black sediment so common and so unpleasant and objectionable in other preparations of this shrub. This is not one of those medicines gotten up by ignorance, to be palmed off upon the credulous. It is prepared by a careful, experienced and conscientious physician, in obedience to the desire of numberless friends in the profession, in the trade, and among the people. **Every bottle is warranted** to contain the full strength of the medicine in its highest state of purity and development, and is superior to any medicine ever prepared from this shrub under any name, or by any person, firm or company.

HUMPHREYS' WITCH-HAZEL is used both as an **external** and an **internal** remedy; both to **apply** as a **lotion** or wash, and to **take** as a **medicine,** and in many cases it is both **taken** and **applied.**

TAKEN INTERNALLY as a medicine, it may be given in doses of even a teaspoonful or more to adults; and to quite young children, to aged persons, or infirm persons, or to those greatly prostrated by sickness, in smaller doses, not only without injury, but with great benefit.

APPLIED EXTERNALLY as a **lotion** or **liniment** for **soreness, lameness,** a **bruise, sprain, strain** or **wrench;** or for a **burn, scald, excoriation** or **swelling,** or where there is **pain, heat,** or **inflammation,**—its action is at once **cooling, soothing,** and **healing,** while it causes no stain or discoloration upon the skin, or upon the finest fabric, or eruption or rash upon the most sensitive surface.

---

# HUMPHREYS' WITCH-HAZEL.

## DISEASES, ACCIDENTS, AND CONDITIONS WHERE IT IS CURATIVE.

THE limits of a small book will hardly suffice to detail even briefly all the valuable uses of a medicine so generally useful as HUMPHREYS' WITCH-HAZEL. Yet some of its more general and specific curative properties may be pointed out, and the scientific explanation or *rationale* of its action given, with the assurance that this medicine has now been in use more than **thirty years,** and its curative power in every particular disease, accident, or condition mentioned, has been **verified** and **confirmed** by multiform and **manifold experience,** and may be implicitly relied upon. The cases of cures, and the concurrent testimony of **Homeopathic, Old School,** and **Eclectic Physicians,** may be found scattered over the pages of current **Medical Literature,** and apply to HUMPHREYS' WITCH-HAZEL with the same force and pertinence as to any other name by which this medicine has been known.

HUMPHREYS' WITCH-HAZEL is the sovereign remedy for all **accidents,** or **injuries** to **man** or **beast** that are within the reach of medicines. These are known specially as **Falls, Blows, Bruises, Contusions, Strains, Sprains, Luxations, Lacerations, Cuts,** or **Incised Wounds, Burns, Scalds, Fractures** and **Dislocations.**

FOR all these conditions, or the results of them, there is no remedy which so perfectly fulfills the conditions of a cure as HUMPHREYS' WITCH-HAZEL; none which so **promptly revives** the **depressed vital action, restores the general and local circulation, allays the pain, dissipates the**

**congestion, prevents inflammation, and restores the healthy action** as HUMPHREYS' WITCH-HAZEL. In thousands of instances the prompt and free application of this medicine has **staunched the bleeding, allayed the pain, removed the congestion, resolved the inflammation** and **promoted the healing** of the most dangerous injury so promptly and magically as to have given it the name of the "MARVEL OF HEALING."

HOW a simple non-poisonous **Vegetable Medicine** should do so much for the prompt relief and cure of serious injuries or grave diseases, is indeed a **marvel.** Yet a scientific and satisfactory explanation is not wanting. The learned and astute Dr. Hering, of Philadelphia, said, and truly, many years ago, when investigating the virtues of WITCH-HAZEL, that it was a union of **Aconite** and **Arnica.** Subsequent observation and experience has fully justified his remark. It has, indeed, the sedative power of **Aconite** in controlling the circulation, arresting the turbulent action of the heart, allaying the heat and removing fever; while it has also the power of **Arnica** in removing soreness and alleviating pain, dissipating congestions, removing engorgements, promoting absorption, and thus dissipating and preventing the evil effects of injuries. Hence, HUMPHREYS' WITCH-HAZEL should be in every **Hospital** and **Infirmary,** in every **Dentist's** and **Doctor's office,** in every **family** or **factory,** in every **stable, shop** or **ship.** It is **the remedy,** always ready for an emergency, **prompt in its action, always reliable, always curative,** doing all that medicine can do.

## HOW TO USE IT FOR ACCIDENTS OR INJURIES.

FOR a **severe fall, shock, blow,** or **contusion,** or **injury.**—The system first suffers, in serious cases, a partial collapse from the result of the shock,—the lips become cold, and face pale, and the entire person is chilled. **Give at once** half a teaspoonful of HUMPHREYS' WITCH-HAZEL, and repeat it every ten or fifteen minutes until the circulation is restored, and the shock passes over. Apply the WITCH-HAZEL freely to the injured parts in full strength, unless the part is torn or lacerated, when it may be reduced one-half with water, and the injured part may then be kept wet with it by repeated applications, or the injury may be properly bound up with a bandage and the WITCH-HAZEL, full strength, frequently applied to the part **through the bandage.** The bandage should be kept wet with the WITCH-HAZEL, and need not be changed for several days. The healing, by **first intention,** will go on beneath the bandage.

FOR a **bruise, contusion, strain,** or **sprain, luxation,** or **wrench.**—These most commonly happen to some joint or more exposed part of the person, and if the patient is faint, give half a teaspoonful internally at once, and bathe the injured part with the WITCH-HAZEL, full strength. Then make a proper compress of three or more thicknesses of linen or cotton cloth, which wet in the WITCH-HAZEL and apply over the injured part, keeping it in place with a bandage. Then keep the part wet with the WITCH-HAZEL, **through the bandage,** which may be kept in place until the injury is cured. If too tight from the swelling of the part, loosen the bandage a trifle, and apply again, keeping it wet with the WITCH-HAZEL. This will **keep down the swelling, heat,** and **inflammation, subdue the pain,** and **promote the healing.**

**BLACK and Blue Spots,** or **Ecchymosis.**—These unsightly discolorations are well-known after every severe injury, and result from the broken or congested vessels and extravasated blood of the part. HUMPHREYS' WITCH-HAZEL, by its power of stimulating absorption, and increasing the capillary circulation, rapidly promotes their disappearance. It is only necessary to frequently bathe the parts with the WITCH-HAZEL, or, when the location admits of it, to lay on a compress kept saturated with the medicine.

**CUTS, Incised,** or **Lacerated Wounds.**—If the wound is yet bleeding, apply the WITCH-HAZEL, full strength, to **arrest** the **hemorrhage.** Bring the edges of the wound together, as neatly as may be, and keep them in place with a proper roller or strap bandage, neatly applied to the part, **and through this,** keep the wound constantly wet with the WITCH-HAZEL. The most severe lacerations have thus been healed, and very serious mutilations and loss of members prevented. If sufficient substance has been left to maintain the circulation, the case thus treated may be safely left to the curative powers of this MARVEL OF HEALING,—HUMPHREYS' WITCH-HAZEL.

**FRACTURES** and **Dislocations** require similar treatment. Give at first half a teaspoonful internally, to allay the sensibility and restore from the shock. Bathe the part with the WITCH-HAZEL freely, until the surgeon arrives and the limb is put in place, or the fracture reduced. Then, from time to time, wet the part, and keep it wet through the bandage. It will rapidly reduce the inflammation, keep down the heat and pain, and promote the healing.

**BURNS** and **Scalds** should be promptly treated with the WITCH-HAZEL. If the injury is only superficial and not extended through the entire skin, lay over the injured part a thin linen or even cotton cloth, which has been wet with the WITCH-HAZEL, and keep this carefully applied over the entire burned surface, so as to exclude the air, and **keep it constantly wet with** WITCH-HAZEL. If the injury has been deeper, destroying the skin so that it hangs in shreds, leaving an extensive raw surface, apply the WITCH-HAZEL in the same way, only diluting it one-third or one-half with water at first, and afterwards using it in full strength. Once per day, the dead parts or shreds may be carefully removed, and the part covered again and kept wet with HUMPHREYS' WITCH-HAZEL until healed. **The first application** relieves the pain and anguish, and the subsequent use keeps down the fever and inflammation, and promotes the healing in the most remarkable manner. **For the Ulcerations,** and **tendency** to **contractions,** consequent upon severe burns, the WITCH-HAZEL OIL is a still more efficient remedy, and being in the form of a salve or ointment, may be simply applied to the raw or ulcerated surface two or three times per day with the most marvelous effect in **healing up the ulcerations** and **preventing** the **hardening** of the **tissues** and **contractions** which are so liable to occur. Slighter forms of **Burns, Scalds,** or **Sunburns, etc.,** require only occasional wetting with the WITCH-HAZEL, say two or three times a day in order to their prompt cure.

**SUNBURNS,** or burning even to peeling of the skin of the face or other parts from exposure to the sun or wind, especially when on the water, are promptly cured by a few applications. Simply bathe freely the face or sunburned part, and repeat the application from time to time every two or three hours. The first application gives relief, and the redness and burning disappear like magic. No hunter or fisherman should go on an excursion without a bottle of HUMPHREYS' WITCH-HAZEL.

**INJURIES** of **Animals,** such as **shoulder strains,** violent **contusions, thrust from a horn, stake,** or **shaft,** often causing terrible lacerations or wounds, find their best remedy in HUMPHREYS' WITCH-HAZEL. In one case, a valuable horse, driven at high speed, was struck by a sleigh-shaft driven violently against him. The point of the shaft struck the lower point of the shoulder, and glancing up beneath the surface a distance of twelve inches, protruded at the top of the shoulder-blade. In the fall and struggle of the two animals, vehicles and men, the shaft was pulled from the terrible wound. It was simply dressed with HUMPHREYS' WITCH-HAZEL, and a compress laid over the entire wound, and kept saturated with the medicine; marvelous to relate, no fever, no sloughing, no lock-jaw, or other bad consequences resulted, and the horse, in a few weeks, was restored without material loss of value.

A YOUNG HORSE ran away, attached to a buggy. In his flight and fall a shaft became broken, and the splinter was driven through one of his feet. Entering just below the fetlock, the broken shaft was driven down and forwards, and protruded several inches out through the sole of the foot. Several sharp blows with a large hammer drove back the inch-thick fragments, and so terrible was the wound, that a veterinary surgeon ordered the animal shot as worthless. The limb was, however, **simply bathed and kept wet with this medicine.** It healed kindly, with no serious malformation, and the horse was restored to service and soundness. **Hundreds of cases,** only varying in extent and severity, have been thus cured by this remedy. In all cases apply the WITCH-HAZEL freely, and, when possible, apply a compress kept in place with a bandage saturated with the WITCH-HAZEL.

**BREAST GALLS, Saddle Galls,** or **Harness Chafings,** are promptly cured by bathing with cold water, and then applying the WITCH-HAZEL three or more times per day.

FOR a **quarter crack, sand crack, quitter,** and especially for **strains** of a tendon, or **lameness,** or **injury** of a **joint.**—Bathe freely with the WITCH-HAZEL, and, when possible, give the animal rest, and apply the compress wet with the medicine. It will keep the part cool, **prevent inflammation,** and rapidly promote the healing.

## HEMORRHAGES, OR BLEEDINGS.

**NEARLY allied to Accidents** are those often terrible occurrences known as **Hemorrhages,** or **Bleedings.** These occur from various sources or organs, and in varying degrees of intensity or danger, but are so often life-inimical and threatening as always to excite the livliest apprehension and alarm. Often a patient is brought to the greatest extremity, and life itself not unfrequently lost for the want of the timely use of a remedy like HUMPHREYS' WITCH-HAZEL. **This medicine is the greatest styptic ever discovered.** It possesses a control over **all Hemorrhages,** from whatever source or from whatever cause, that is **perfectly marvelous,** and could scarcely be credited were the testimony less positive or less overwhelming. Its power over hemorrhages seems three-fold,—first, to lessen the action of the heart, hence, the **force of the circulation**: next, to modify and **control the capillary circulation,** whether of the **mucous membrane** or the **pulmonary tissue,** and, finally, its power of **increasing the coagulability** of the blood. Hence, we account for the thousands of **cures of hemorrhages** reported in medicine, and known among the people, by this remedy. Hence it happens that whenever taken, or applied for, **bleeding from a cut,** or **laceration,** or **injury,** or from the **gums** by the extraction of a **tooth,** or from the **nose,** the **throat,** or the **lungs** or **bronchiæ,** from the **stomach,** from the **womb,** or from **Piles,** or even in that most intractable condition, the **Hemorrhagic Diathesis** is controlled in the most **wonderful manner** by the benign action of this remedy.

**HEMORRHAGE** from the **nose** rarely assumes a severe or dangerous form except when in connection with a dissolute condition of the blood, such as occurs in consumptive or scorbutic subjects, or in typhus fevers, purpurea or in connection with the hemorrhagic diathesis. There are a vast number of cases recorded in Medicine, either of habitual nose-bleed, or when merely accidental, which have been cured by this remedy, and so prompt and decided its action, as to leave nothing more to be desired. Simple cases will be promptly cured by taking ten drops of HUMPHREYS' WITCH-HAZEL internally, and laying a cloth wet with it across the bridge of the nose, after bathing the forehead and nose with it. In more severe cases, half a teaspoonful of the medicine may be put into half a common glass of water, and of this dilution a spoonful may be given every fifteen minutes. The WITCH-HAZEL may be thrown up the bleeding nostril, with a small syringe, or in some cases the nostrils may be plugged with lint, saturated with the medicine.

**BLEEDING from the gums,** or from having had teeth extracted.—These hemorrhages are rarely troublesome, except in connection with a scorbutic, or hemorrhagic diathesis. In either case the WITCH-HAZEL is perfectly adapted. For bleeding from the mouth or gums, simply rinse the mouth from time to time with the WITCH-HAZEL, which may be afterwards repeated four or more times per day to heal up the gums. **After a tooth has been extracted,** and the first mouthful of blood been discharged, always rinse the mouth with the WITCH-HAZEL. This may be repeated every few minutes until the bleeding is arrested.

## BLEEDING OR HEMORRHAGE FROM THE LUNGS.

THIS truly formidable condition is controlled and cured by no medicine so completely and perfectly as by HUMPHREYS' WITCH-HAZEL. The hemorrhage may arise from congestion and the rupture of minute, or even more considerable blood-vessels, or from congestion and exudation from minute capillaries, or from the progress of tuburcular disease, and the dissolute condition of the blood and relaxed pulmonary capillaries.

IN all these conditions the hemorrhage falls within the immediate curative action of this remedy. Hence it is not surprising to find the large number of cases of cures by this medicine recorded in medical literature. In one case, a stout, heavy man, after experiencing for a day or two a kind of fullness and oppression in the chest, after a slight cough found himself spitting up blood by the mouthful. He soon became weak, faint, and prostrated, and after the use of several remedies, resorted, by the advice of a friend, to the WITCH-HAZEL. A dose of ten drops was given every fifteen minutes, after which the bleeding gradually ceased, and never returned again. Dr. Payne reports the case of a young lady of sixteen, tall, slender, pale skin, blue eyes, light hair, who was attacked by spitting of blood without premonitory symptoms. The bleeding commenced with a slight hack, and continued with scarce a moment's intermission for nearly an hour. The blood seemed to come into the mouth without effort, and to flow from a point some ten inches below the right clavicle. Several remedies were given without effect, when four drops of the WITCH-HAZEL, in half a glass of water, of which a spoonful was given with immediate relief, and the bleeding did not return again. A young gentleman of 26, whose health had been impaired in the army, was attacked with repeated and profuse hemorrhage from the lungs. These attacks came at intervals of from three to six months, and were characterized by profuse discharge of blood. It came without effort, or with a slight hack, and the patient sat without speaking or moving, with pale, anxious countenance, saturating napkin after napkin with darkish, frothy blood, until the system was perfectly exsanguined, or seemingly bloodless. Every known remedy was exhausted, with only temporary relief, when the WITCH-HAZEL was resorted to. Half a teaspoonful was mixed in half a glass of water, of which a spoonful was given every fifteen minutes, with prompt relief of the bleeding. A compress saturated with the medicine was laid over the chest, and worn at night when the chest felt full and heavy, under which treatment the hemorrhage never returned. These three typical cases, out of many that might be given, are sufficient to show the marvelous control of this medicine over pulmonary hemorrhages. The method of application is sufficiently indicated. Half a teaspoonful of the medicine may be mixed in a common tumbler half full of water, and of this solution a teaspoonful may be given every fifteen or thirty minutes until relieved, then every two or three hours to prevent a return. If the chest is hot or sore, saturate a cloth with HUMPHREYS' WITCH-HAZEL, and lay on over the affected place, the whole covered with a dry flannel to protect the clothing.

**VOMITING of Blood, Bleeding from the Stomach, Hematemesis, profuse Bloody Stools of dark thick blood.—Melæna, Bleeding from the Stomach,** or other portions of the intestinal track, may arise from abdominal congestion, or from a ruptured vessel, or from ulceration even when of a cancerous nature, or from Piles, but in many cases will be found in connection with a dissolute condition of the blood. In every case the condition falls within the curative action of the WITCH-HAZEL, and for which it will be found a sovereign remedy. There are numerous cases on record of its efficient action under various and far different modifications of this condition. KING' states that it is curative in **Hematemesis** and has cured by merely a decoction of the bark, a spoonful every three hours. PRESTON has cured bleeding with this remedy when it arose from cancerous ulceration, as well as that from mechanical congestion of the portal circulation. GREEN reports a severe case of melæna attended with profuse discharge of dark clotted blood, the stools filling a large-sized chamber. The patient had a former but less severe attack a week previous. The case was successfully treated with the WITCH-HAZEL and cured. BELCHER reports a severe case of vomiting and purging of blood cured by this remedy. In another case, a young man in the last stages of typhus abdominalis was attacked with profuse exhausting stools of dark, grumous blood, so that his life was fast ebbing away, when he was given this medicine, fifteen drops every hour, with prompt relief, and made a final recovery. DR. PRATT reports a similar case of intestinal hemorrhage, occuring in the course of typhoid fever, when stools of pure blood were repeated every fifteen minutes, and at least two quarts had been passed before the patient was visited, and which was cured by the mother tincture of the WITCH-HAZEL, given at first every ten minutes, and afterwards at intervals of an hour. The directions may be varied to suit individual cases, but in general put a large spoonful of HUMPHREYS' WITCH-HAZEL in a glass half-filled with water, of which give a large spoonful every fifteen, thirty or sixty minutes, according to the urgency of the case, and then two or three times a day to prevent a return.

**HEMATURIA, or Bloody Urine,** falls directly within the curative action of this remedy, and numerous cases are reported as cured by it, in current medical literature. It is equally efficient whether the hemorrhage is renal, visical, or urethral. The WITCH-HAZEL should be given in doses of ten or fifteen drops, and repeated every two or three hours for any form of bloody urination, and may be fully relied upon for a cure.

**HEMORRHAGE from the Uterus, Flooding, Metrorrhagia.**—The most dangerous forms of this affection arise from premature delivery, or abortion in consequence of severe injury, and are hence brought within the curative action of this remedy. The WITCH-HAZEL will prove effectual in all similar cases, and may also be given with great benefit in all cases of too profuse and too long-lasting menses. For flooding, give half a teaspoonful every fifteen minutes until an impression is made, and then at longer intervals. **For too profuse menses** give ten drops three times per day during the period. **Hemorrhage from Piles, Bleeding Piles.**—The specific action of the WITCH-HAZEL over venous hemorrhages points unmistakably to its cure of bleeding Piles, and affords an explanation of its wonderful cures and great reputation in this connection.

**BLEEDING Piles, Blind Piles, Hemorrhoids,** in their various stages of development and degree, form the especial pathological condition for the specific action of HUMPHREYS' WITCH-HAZEL. **Piles** are always the result of abdominal venous congestion, and obstruction of the portal circulation. From this results venous engorgements, local swellings, formation of tumors, and subsequent distress, pain in the back, formations of hemorrhoidal growths, and frequent hemorrhage. **No remedy so perfectly controls, or so permanently removes this entire condition** as HUMPHREYS'

WITCH-HAZEL. Taken internally, and applied, if the piles are external, in the form of a lotion, or of the WITCH-HAZEL OIL, or even injected in cases of internal piles, the pain and distress are relieved, the bleeding arrested, the tumors become flaccid, and shrink away, and gradually disappear, and a permanent cure is accomplished. The number of cases recorded in current medical literature, or known among the people, as cured by this remedy in its various forms, is almost innumerable. Every medical writer or physician who has had occasion to speak of WITCH-HAZEL, praises its efficacy in the cure of Piles. It has been used in this disease from the earliest settlement of the country, and it is quite probable the knowledge of its earlier use was obtained from the Indians. DRS. KING, HALL, HERING, OKIE, FREEMAN, DAVIDSON, CHASE, and many others, all bear concurrent testimony of its great value. **Cases of Piles,** that have resisted all other methods of cure and medicine, and where the patients have been incapacitated for business for years, have been cured permanently by this remedy. A sinewy man of florid face and sanguine temperament, a Merchant formerly doing business in New York, had been a martyr to piles for thirty years, had lost immense amounts of blood, and twice been operated upon for Piles, and finally was obliged to abandon his business in consequence of the disease. He was readily cured by the use of this medicine taken and applied in connection with the Homeopathic medicine. **The Book** might be filled with the record of cases of **Piles** cured by this remedy. It is, if possible, more especially curative where the piles bleed frequently, and are attended with a sense of soreness, excoriation, or burning, and pain in the back; but **every case of Piles, however constituted,** will be relieved by it. If the piles are external, bathe the parts and apply a cloth saturated with the WITCH-HAZEL, and kept in place by a bandage passing around the loins, and a tail-piece passing down over the part, and brought up and secured in front; also take a half teaspoonful three or four times per day. For obstinate internal piles inject an ounce at night on retiring to rest and retain it if possible, or still better, apply the WITCH-HAZEL OIL. **The cure is infallible.**

**RHEUMATISM and Rheumatic Pains, Lameness, Soreness.**—This remedy has most specific action in **Rheumatism** and **Rheumatic pains,** occurring in various parts of the body or limbs. **Pains** and **Lameness in the wrist, arm** or **shoulder, pain** or **stiffness of the neck,** or of the **hips, knee** or the **ankle** or **foot,** all fall within the range of its curative action. This is true, whether the affection arise from **recent cold, exposure, overwork** or **strain.** In all these cases, simply bathing the parts with HUMPHREYS' WITCH-HAZEL two or three times per day, will promptly relieve the pain and soreness and restore the part to health. Half a teaspoonful may also be taken internally every two hours.

**INFLAMMATORY** or **Acute Rheumatism,** attended with **heat, swelling, pain** and **lameness** of one or several joints, requires for its prompt cure the action of the specific Homeopathic Medicine internally, and the application of the WITCH-HAZEL. It should be applied freely to the **swelled, lame** or **suffering part,** and a cloth wet in the medicine kept applied to it. The soreness, lameness and pain will be speedily allayed and a cure promptly attained. It is the best application that can be made as testified by large experience.

**LUMBAGO,** or **Crick in the Back,** is also one of those troublesome Rheumatic affections promptly cured by this remedy. It sometimes comes on suddenly from a chill, a false step, a wound, a strain or from overwork, and for a time holds the patient as in a vice. Take half a spoonful of the WITCH-HAZEL internally and repeat it every hour, and bathe the part with it, or even lay on a cloth saturated with the medicine, over which a dry flannel is placed to protect the clothing, and the relief will be prompt and permanent.

**NEURALGIA** is sometimes so closely allied to Rheumatism, that it is difficult to form the line of demarkation. However this may be, it is well-known that HUMPHREYS' WITCH-HAZEL has prompt control over a large class of these affections. **Pains in the face,** along the side of the head or neck, are promptly cured by freely bathing the affected part, or applying the saturated cloth to the place.

**TOOTHACHE,** either of **Neuralgic** or **Rheumatic origin,** or **arising from a cold,** or the **irritation** of **decayed teeth,** is promptly cured by this remedy. There is often heat and swelling of the gums or surrounding tissues, and in children it is often excited by cold, or the production of new teeth. In all cases of **Toothache,** bathe the face on the side of the affected tooth with the WITCH-HAZEL and take some in the mouth, and hold it on that side—repeating the same as occasion requires. The relief will be prompt. Often, the cloth wet with WITCH-HAZEL, laid over the part, gives a quiet night's rest, with entire subsidence of the pain.

**SWELLED FACE.**—Often in consequence of **Toothache,** and sometimes from **exposure** or **cold,** or of **Rheumatic origin,** the face or cheek of one side becomes swelled, and red or pale, attended with more or less of pain. The WITCH-HAZEL is the natural specific; bathe the part freely with it, and then saturate a cloth and lay on over the part, covering with a dry handerchief, taking ten or fifteen drops of the medicine internally every two hours, and the relief will be prompt. The heat, pain and anguish will disappear, the swelling abate, and the entire affection pass off like magic, leaving not a trace behind.

**SORE THROAT** or **Quinsy.**—HUMPHREYS' WITCH-HAZEL is a very common, and very effectual remedy for Sore Throats, and all the more so because it can be so readily and directly applied to the suffering part;

applied early to the neck or throat by means of a cloth saturated with the medicine, and by a gargle to the suffering part, the inflammation will be dispersed without suppuration; or applied in the same manner at any stage, it relieves the pain, reduces the swelling and tends to rapid restoration, and subsidence of the inflammation and soreness. Persons subject to **Quinsy** should never be without this remedy. Using it in time, they will dissipate the disease without suppuration, and its habitual use, as occasion requires, will invigorate and change the nutrition of the part so as to destroy the predisposition to the disease, as the experience of hundreds can testify.

**SORE Eyes, Inflamed Eyes or Eye-lids.** For chronic or specific forms of **Ophthalmy**, the WITCH-HAZEL cannot be regarded as the special cure, yet there are many forms of simple Sore Eyes, or Eye-lids, attended with **redness, swellings, heat** and **pain,** where a lotion made by putting one part of the WITCH-HAZEL with three parts of soft water, and bathing the eyes frequently with it, will be sovereign benefit, and will promptly control and ultimately cure it. It is especially efficient when the eye-ball **is red,** or **full of red injected vessels,** or when, in consequence of severe cough, or a strain, or injury, the eye-ball is redwith extravasated blood. In all cases it forms a soothing curative lotion, and for simple inflamed, sore, or congested eyes, or eyelids is invaluable.

**EARACHE** is one of those distressing and frequently recurring affections, of children or adults, which is promptly controlled by this medicine, simply wetting a pledget of cotton or lint with the WITCH-HAZEL and inserting it in the affected ear will promptly relieve. **Inflammation of the Internal Ear** is a still more painful and dangerous disease. For its cure apply the lint as above and wet a compress with the WITCH-HAZEL and keep it applied to the face and ear affected. It will promptly modify and control this most painful affection.

**CATARRH.** This remedy, under various names, has been largely used for the cure of **Catarrh,** and for most forms it is truly a specific. As an injection for the nose in old, obstinate Catarrh, or when there is profuse or offensive discharge, it can hardly be excelled. It should be diluted three parts to one with pure water, and then injected or thrown up the nostril with a small nasal syringe, the bulb of rubber and the point of hard rubber or glass, and enlarged at the end to fit the nostril, so that the medicine may be repeatedly injected and returned again into the instrument without inconvenience or wetting the face or clothes; used in this manner the WITCH-HAZEL will not fail to give satisfaction in the most obstinate cases of Catarrh. (Price $1.50.)

EVERY **Dentist's Office** should be supplied with HUMPHREYS' WITCH-HAZEL. Aside from its value in the hemorrhage incident to the extracting of teeth, and which in subjects of **Hemorrhagic Diathesis** may become dangerous or even fatal, **every operation upon the mouth or teeth** will be wonderfully facilitated in the healing by the use of this medicine. The **bleeding and soreness of the gums,** the **strained, sore, excoriated feeling of the mouth and face,** and the tenderness or soreness of the teeth operated upon, are all wonderfully relieved and soothed by simply rinsing the mouth in HUMPHREYS' WITCH-HAZEL. No dentist who has once experienced its benign effect will consent to be without it in his office. See also **Bleeding from the Gums.**

PAINS, **Stitches or Soreness and Tightness of the Chest.** These obscure, sometimes rheumatic and sometimes congestive, pains in the chest are promptly relieved by HUMPHREYS' WITCH-HAZEL, taking half a teaspoonful three or four times per day.

BOILS, **Furuncles, Hot Swellings, and Carbuncles.** All forms of hot or painful inflammatory swellings are treated with great success by this remedy. So soon as a swelling is perceived or pain manifested, HUMPHREYS' WITCH-HAZEL should be applied. It will often arrest further progress and discuss them. In case of **boils, hot swellings,** or **carbuncles,** cover the swelling with lint, saturated with the medicine; it will relieve the pain and heat, and limit the extension of the suppurative process, and promote the healing.

TUMORS **or Cold Swellings.** Some very remarkable cures have been made by this medicine of **Abdominal Tumors.** When it is remembered how frequently such tumors occur, and how difficult is the cure except by the most terrible surgical operation, the importance of obtaining a cure by the use of a simple medicine will be recognized. A middle-aged lady, Madam ——, of dark complexion and vigorous health, gradually was made aware of the presence of a tumor in the lower left portion of the abdomen. When first noticed it was the size of one's fist, with a corresponding increase of the entire abdomen, and in the course of six months it had attained the size of a child's head, filling and distending the entire abdominal cavity, and seriously interfering with her health. She consulted several of the most eminent of the profession of New York, among others Drs. Simms and Parker. The diagnosis was unquestioned and the advice was to resort to an operation as the only prospect of recovery. By advice of a physician, she commenced the use of this medicine, wearing a compress wet with it over the abdomen, and taking a teaspoonful three times per day, and using it as a vaginal injection. To her great delight there was prompt relief of the pain, distress, and abdominal distension, and in less than six months the tumor had diminished more than one-half, and the patient had fully regained her vigor. At the end of a year, the tumor could be scarcely felt, and the patient considered herself well, though still using the medicine. This is most remarkable. **Of the fact,** there is no dispute. Is this so, that these abdominal or ovarian tumors, the dread of the profession, are the result of congestion of the abdominal (portal) circulation, and that the removal of this engorgement simply withdraws the nutrition, and thus causes the absorption of these formidable growths? It would seem so. One who has carefully studied the effect of this medicine is driven to this conclusion.

**DISEASES of the Ovaries, Congestion, Inflammation, Enlargement.—** This remedy has a very decided and positive action in various forms of ovarian diseases, as corroborated by its action as above mentioned. The earlier observers of its action bear testimony of its efficacy. Dr. LUDLAM has found it efficacious in several cases of ovarian diseases, accompanied with **pain, swelling,** and **tenderness** of the ovarian region. Dr. OKIE used it as a cure for ovarian disease following an injury, where there was violent pain in and about the ovary, and, at times, soreness over the entire abdomen, and extreme sensibility of all the associated organs and regions, irregular menses, and retention of the urine. The case was cured by this medicine, used as a vaginal injection and as an application. It has been used with success in numerous similar cases, attended with **pain, tenderness,** and **distress** in the ovarian region. For all such cases use a vaginal injection of HUMPHREYS' WITCH-HAZEL, diluted one-half with water; apply the wet compress to the part, and take fifteen drops four times per day. The relief will be speedy, and the result every way gratifying.

**MENSTRUAL Irregularities, Painful, Too Profuse,** or **Vicarious Menstruation.**—Painful menses are often immediately relieved by taking half a spooful. The pain and distress is relieved, and the discharge becomes natural. In like manner, when the flow has lasted **too long** and been **too profuse,** and especially if dark and thick, the use of half a spoonful of WITCH-HAZEL, morning and night, will regulate and arrest the drain. **In Vicarious Menses,** or where, instead of the monthly flow, there appears a bleeding from the nose, lungs, or other part, the action of this remedy cannot be too highly praised. Ten drops of HUMPHREYS' WITCH-HAZEL, taken every one, two, or three hours, according to the urgency of the case, promptly arrests the hemorrhage, and promotes the natural discharge. Numerous successful cases of this nature are on record.

**ULCERATION.**—This condition, so common and yet so often obstinate, yields to the application of this mild remedy in a manner approached by no other medicine. Thousands of ladies are martyrs to ulceration of the womb, with various accessories—bearing down, enlargement, etc.—and hundreds rejoice that they first made the acquaintance of this medicine. Even when the ulceration has become chronic, with tendency to schirrhus degeneration of the part, the free application of the WITCH-HAZEL has been found to work wonders. It should be applied daily two or three times, as an injection—one part of the WITCH-HAZEL to two parts of water—by means of a vaginal syringe. Humphreys' New Female Syringe is the best, as it is more convenient, allows a more complete application of the medicine to the parts, and is more economical in the use of the fluid. (Price $2.00.)

**LEUCORRHEA,** or **Whites,** is another of those troublesome forms of disease which finds a true curative in HUMPHREYS' WITCH-HAZEL, applied as an injection, the same as recommended for ulceration. It tones up the mucous membrane, and gives strength to the entire system, while it promptly arrests and cures the discharge. This is more especially true in regard to vaginal **Leucorrhea,** but is true also of uterine **Leucorrhea,** from the sympathetic action of the medicine. There are numerous physicians whose practice has been largely built up from their success in curing various forms of **Female Weakness** with this medicine, used under various names and forms.

**INFLAMED** or **Gathered Breast** should be treated with WITCH-HAZEL. As soon as there is pain in the breast or a chill or reddish blush (erysipelatous) is noticed, apply a cloth wet in the WITCH-HAZEL, which renew as often as it gets dry or heated, over which place a fold of dry flannel to protect the clothing. This will often arrest the inflammatory progress altogether, and in any event, will relieve the heat and pain, or limit the suppurative process.

**EXCORIATED** or **Sore Nipples** may be cured, or the soreness prevented, by bathing them with the WITCH-HAZEL **before** and **after** the child has nursed. It should be diluted one-half with soft water.

**EXCORIATIONS,** or **soreness,** or **chafing** of infants, will be prevented, or when present, will be cured by applying the WITCH-HAZEL to the part. Either add an ounce of the WITCH-HAZEL to the water in which the child is bathed—or, after bathing, apply the WITCH-HAZEL, diluted one-half with water, to the part, after which dry the part as usual.

**KIDNEY Complaints.**—There are various forms of renal disease for which this medicine is curative. **Pain** in the region of the Kidneys or small of the back, and **painful, frequent** or **scalding urination,** are among the symptoms which are promptly removed by its use. It is also very useful in cases of **Strangury, with painful scalding,** or **incontinence.**

GRAVEL, or **Renal Calculi,** attended with **painful frequent urging** or **incontinence.** Half a spoonful three times per day has cured several old and very obstinate cases.

STINGS of **Insects, Mosquitoes, Bees, or Spiders.**—The results of these bites or stings are promptly controlled and removed by the application of HUMPHREYS' WITCH-HAZEL. Simply bathe the part with the remedy, and repeat the application from time to time until the pain and swelling are relieved. It acts like magic for mosquito bites. For severe bee or hornet stings, saturate a cloth with the medicine and lay over the part. The cure is prompt and certain. A few applications remove every trace of mosquito bites.

CHAPPED **Hands.**—Often, especially in Winter, or in rough cold weather, or from exposure, and especially in some persons, the hands become rough, chapped or even sore or readily bleeding. A WITCH-HAZEL bath is the best remedy. Add a spoonful to a pint of water, with which bathe freely. The soreness and roughness will be removed, and the skin softened and healed.

AFFECTIONS **of the Veins.**—From the control which this remedy has over the venous circulation, might be inferred its ability to cure various diseases of the veins. This presumption has been abundantly verified by experience, and practitioners have found this the most reliable remedy known for **inflammation of the Veins (Phlebitis), engorged** or **varicose veins,** and all those morbid conditions thence arising.

INFLAMMATION **of the Veins.**—There are several cases recorded of prompt cures of this disease by this remedy. Dr. BARNES cured a case of "inflammation of the femoral vein, with an erysipelatous spot over the vein, near the groin, and spreading over half the thigh, swelling of the entire leg and foot, heat and pale appearance of the limb." Dr. ROBINSON cured a case attended with great pain in the right leg, from the knee to the hip; leg swelled and sensitive; veins hard, knotted, swollen, and painful; skin erysipelatous; abdominal veins hard like cords, red and painful. These cases are sufficient to show its specific action. The WITCH-HAZEL should be taken in doses of ten drops, repeated every two hours, and the medicine applied over the inflamed surface by means of a cloth saturated with it, and renewed from time to time as it becomes hot or dry.

MILK **Leg,** or **Phlegmasia Alba Dolens,** being essentially a phlebitis, inflammation of the uterine veins, falls directly within the curative action of this remedy. Several physicians—among them Dr. OKIE—having had large experience with it, highly extol it in this disease, as being by far the most **prompt, specific** and **reliable remedy** known. It is not only applicable to those cases attended with pain, lameness, tenderness, and swelling of the limb, but also to more chronic cases where the disease has left behind it a lameness and frequently-recurring swelling of the limb. Acute cases should be treated the same as an acute Phlebitis (see above), and chronic cases should have the limb bathed in WITCH-HAZEL two or three times per day, and fifteen drops also taken at the same time. The effect will be prompt and permanent.

**VARICOSE Veins.**—The practitioner will be at no loss to infer that the WITCH-HAZEL is the **true specific** for varicose veins; and will not be surprised to learn how uniform is the testimony concerning it. Dr. PRESTON affirms that he has himself used it in more than fifty cases without a single failure. Others have used it as extensively with like success, so that these unsightly knotted bluish veins, often the size of a finger, may now be regarded as reduceable by this comparatively simple medicine. The plan is simple; lay a cloth over the enlarged veins or over the whole limb, saturated with the WITCH-HAZEL, over which turn an **elastic bandage** (rubber stocking) from the arch of the foot up and over the affected part. Renew the cloth night and morning, taking also fifteen drops of the medicine. The rapid relief and diminution of the unsightly veins is something wonderful.

**VARICOCELE.**—This condition — enlargement and dilation of the spermatic veins—can be reduced and cured by means of the WITCH-HAZEL, used in a similar manner. Apply a compress saturated with the medicine, and kept in place by a suspensory bandage, and renew the application daily. Numerous cases have been cured.

**ULCERS, Old Sores.**—These affections are often formidable, and sometimes life long companions. They usually appear in consequence of fever or a depraved condition of the blood, intimately connected with venus congestion. **Superficial ulcers of the legs** are almost invariably connected with varicose veins. They should be dressed daily with WITCH-HAZEL, diluted one-half with water, and then apply a compress wet with the same and over the whole, the elastic stocking. Common ulcers of the legs will thus be soon cured. **Deep, foul, painful, spreading ulcers** require a dressing of lint, saturated with the WITCH-HAZEL, applied over the part, and removed as often as the dressing becomes dry or hot, and the limb or part kept up and at rest for a speedy healing.

**FELON, Panaris.**—These affections are known as deep-seated inflammations, occurring along or at the end of the finger, beneath the nail, or beneath a tendon, and by the severe pain and sometimes extensive ulceration of the part. The early use of the WITCH-HAZEL, binding up the part in a saturated cloth, renewing the same when it becomes dry or heated, frequently arrests the disease; and kept applied in any stage, it limits the inflammation, mitigates the pain, and promotes the healing.

**CORNS and Bunions.**—These should be soaked in warm water, and then pared down as far as the quick will permit. Then apply the WITCH-

HAZEL, full strength, at night, with a wet compress. The soreness will be at once relieved, and the frequent application of the remedy will cure this source of annoyance.

**SORE Feet.**—Some persons have habitually sensitive feet, so as to cause them great annoyance, in case of severe or sometimes only moderate usage. Simply bathe the feet every night and morning; and after wiping them dry, wet them with the WITCH-HAZEL, or use a bath of diluted WITCH-HAZEL (one ounce to a quart of water). It will promptly relieve and soon cure the most obstinate cases.

**CHILBLAINS** are too well-known to require a description. The small, red, itching and burning points along the heels or soles of the feet will be at once relieved by bathing them at night with HUMPHREYS' WITCH-HAZEL.

**FROSTED Parts,** after having been treated in the usual manner by snow or in water, will be relieved and the cure promoted by bathing them frequently with HUMPHREYS' WITCH-HAZEL.

**EXCORIATIONS, Soreness,** or **Blisters** of the hands or feet, or other parts of the body, in consequence of rowing, driving, ball-playing, or other labor or exposure, are promptly relieved by bathing the injured surface with the WITCH-HAZEL, repeating the application two or three times per day.

**DIARRHEA.**—Ten or fifteen drops taken in a spoonful of water, is a good remedy for a mucous diarrhea or looseness of the bowels. For **Chronic Diarrhea,** half a spoonful, three times a day, has cured many cases.

**DYSENTERY.** This is a valuable remedy in some forms of Dysentery, when the stools are large and consist mostly of **black grumous blood,** or **blood** and **mucous.** It may be given ten drops on a bit of sugar, and a large spoonful mixed in a teacupful of thin starch, used as an injection.

**AS a Toilet Article**—HUMPHREYS' WITCH-HAZEL cannot be excelled. A tablespoonful mixed in the usual cup of shaving water, wonderfully softens the lather, and takes away the **soreness, roughness, smarting** and sense of **excoriation,** so common after shaving, while it heals up any **cut, eruption** or **pimple** which may have been exposed.

**A WITCH-HAZEL bath** is a luxury.—A small quantity, an ounce, or less, added to the bowl of water, wonderfully softens the water and revives, invigorates, and refreshes the face or person, and improves the complexion to a degree inconceivable to those who have not given it a trial. PRICE.—6 oz. Bottles, 50 cts.; Pints, $1.00; Quarts, $1.75. Each bottle contains full quantity named. Sold by all Dealers.

# LIST OF HUMPHREYS' HOMEOPATHIC SPECIFICS

## FOR FAMILY USE.

---

**Prices of Single Boxes and Vials, with Directions.**

| No. | | | Boxes. | Vials. |
|---|---|---|---|---|
| 1 | Cures | **Fevers,** Congestions, Inflammations, Heat, Pain, Restlessness | $ 25 | $0 50 |
| 2 | " | **Worm Fever,** Worm Colic, Voracious Appetite | 25 | 50 |
| 3 | " | **Colic,** Teething, Crying and Wakefulness of Infants | 25 | 50 |
| 4 | " | **Diarrhœa** of Children or Adults, Cholera Infantum | 25 | 50 |
| 5 | " | **Dysentery** or Bloody Flux, Gripings, Bilious Colic | 25 | 50 |
| 6 | " | **Cholera,** Cholera Morbus, Nausea, Vomiting | 25 | 50 |
| 7 | " | **Coughs,** Colds, Hoarseness, Bronchitis, Influenza | 25 | 50 |
| 8 | " | **Toothache,** Faceache, Neuralgia, Tic Douloureux | 25 | 50 |
| 9 | " | **Headache,** Sick Headache, Vertigo, Congestion | 25 | 50 |
| 10 | " | **Dyspepsia,** Weak, Acid or Deranged Stomach, Costiveness | 25 | 50 |
| 11 | " | **Suppressed Menses,** or Scanty, or Painful, or Delaying | 25 | 50 |
| 12 | " | **Leucorrhœa** or **Whites,** Bearing Down, Profuse Menses | 25 | 50 |
| 13 | " | **Croup,** Hoarse, Croupy Cough, Difficult Breathing | 25 | 50 |
| 14 | " | **Salt Rheum,** Eruptions, Erysipelas, Scald Head | 25 | 50 |
| 15 | " | **Rheumatism,** Pain in the Chest, Back, Side, or Limbs | 25 | 50 |
| 16 | " | **Fever and Ague,** Intermittent Fever, Dumb Ague | 50 | 50 |
| 17 | " | **Piles,** Internal or External, Blind or Bleeding | 50 | 50 |
| 18 | " | **Ophthalmia,** Weak or Inflamed Eyes or Eyelids | 50 | 50 |
| 19 | " | **Catarrh,** Acute or Chronic, Dry or Flowing | 50 | 50 |
| 20 | " | **Hooping Cough,** Shortening and Palliating it | 50 | 50 |
| 21 | " | **Asthma,** Oppressed, Difficult, Labored Breathing | 50 | 50 |
| 22 | " | **Ear Discharges,** Noise in the Head, Difficult Hearing | 50 | 50 |
| 23 | " | **Scrofula,** Enlarged Glands, Swelling and Ulcers | 50 | 50 |
| 24 | " | **General Debility,** Physical or General Weakness | 50 | 50 |
| 25 | " | **Dropsy,** Fluid Accumulations, Tumid Swellings | 50 | 50 |
| 26 | " | **Sea-Sickness,** Prostration, Vertigo, Nausea, Vomiting | 50 | 50 |
| 27 | " | **Urinary Diseases,** Gravel, Renal Calculi | 50 | 50 |
| 28 | " | **Nervous Debility,** Involuntary Discharges, Seminal Weakness, Results of Excess or Evil Habits | 1 00 | 1 00 |
| 29 | " | **Sore Mouth,** or Canker of Adults and Children | 50 | 50 |
| 30 | " | **Urinary Incontinence,** Wetting the Bed, too Frequent, Scalding, or Painful Urination | 50 | 50 |
| 31 | " | **Painful Menses,** Pressure or Spasms, Pruritis | 50 | 50 |
| 32 | " | **Change of Life,** Irregularities, Flushes, Palpitations, and Disease of the Heart | 1 00 | 1 00 |
| 33 | " | **Epilepsy and Spasms,** Chorea or St. Vitus' Dance | 1 00 | 1 00 |
| 34 | " | **Diphtheria,** Ulcerated or Malignant Sore Throat | 50 | 50 |
| 35 | " | **Chronic Congestions,** Habitual Headaches | 50 | 50 |

| | |
|---|---|
| Six SMALL 25c. boxes, with directions | 1 25 |
| Six LARGE 50c. boxes or vials, with directions | 2 50 |
| Six " $1.00 " " | 5 00 |

# LIST OF FAMILY CASES.

| No. | | |
|---|---|---|
| 1. | With **35 Three-Drachm Vials,** ROSEWOOD CASE, containing entire list of 35 numbered Specifics and HUMPHREYS' HOMEOPATHIC MENTOR | $12 00 |
| 2. | With **35 Three-Drachm Vials,** MOROCCO CASE, and Manual of Directions | 10 00 |
| 3. | With **28 Three-Drachm Vials,** MOROCCO CASE and Manual | 8 00 |
| 4. | With **20 Three-Drachm Vials,** MOROCCO CASE and Manual | 6 00 |
| 5. | With **20 Three-Drachm Vials,** PAPER CASE and Manual | 5 00 |

## POCKET CASES.

| | | |
|---|---|---|
| 6. | With **16 Four-Drachm Vials,** RUSSIA LEATHER (double flat), and HUMPHREYS' HOMEOPATHIC MENTOR | $10 00 |
| 7. | With **20 Three-Drachm Vials,** TURKEY MOROCCO or RUSSIA LEATHER (double flat), velvet lined, and Manual | 8 00 |
| 8. | With **10 Three-Drachm Vials** and Manual | 3 50 |
| 9. | With **6 Three-Drachm Vials** and Manual | 2 50 |
| 10. | With **10 One-Drachm Vials** and Manual | 2 00 |

## EXTRA CASES.

| | | |
|---|---|---|
| 11. | With **40 1-oz. Glass-stopper Bottles,** ROSEWOOD CASE, and HUMPHREYS' HOMEOPATHIC MENTOR | $30 00 |
| 12. | With **35 1-oz. Glass-stopper Bottles,** ROSEWOOD CASE and MENTOR. | 25 00 |
| 13. | With **35 1-oz. Vials,** ROSEWOOD CASE and MENTOR | 20 00 |
| 14. | With **12 1-oz. Bottles,** WALNUT CASE and MENTOR | 9 00 |
| | Or, with Manual | 8 00 |
| 15. | With **48 1-oz. Glass-stopper Bottles,** ROSEWOOD CASE, MENTOR, Veterinary and Cholera Manuals | 40 00 |
| MENTOR, with CASE | | 1 50 |

## Asiatic Cholera Specifics (in fluid.)

| | |
|---|---|
| CASES FOR FAMILIES (three large 1 oz. vials), in morocco, with Manual of Directions, containing description of Cholera, its statistics, preventive and curative treatment | $5 00 |
| POCKET CASES, in morocco, for travellers, single persons (3 drachm vials) | 3 00 |
| SINGLE BOTTLES, with directions ... each | 1 00 |

SINGLE VIALS, for replenishing—3 drachms, 75 cents ; 1 ounce, $1.25

## Humphreys' Homeopathic Specifics sent Free by Mail or Express.

These Remedies are sent free to any address on receipt of the price. Thus any person may obtain them—if not at the druggists, then through the nearest Post-office, taking care to send a MONEY ORDER OR REGISTERED LETTER, for safety. If in making an order for a 35, 28, or 20 vial case, some of the kinds or numbers in the list are not wanted, they may be omitted, and DUPLICATES OF THE SAME PRICE may be ordered, so as to make up a case of the kinds desired. This privilege not extending, however, to more than to three of any one kind, and to the numbers 28, 32 and 33 not at all. **All orders for Medicines** should be addressed to

Humphreys' Homeopathic Medicine Co.,

562 BROADWAY, NEW YORK.

# HUMPHREYS' HOMEOPATHIC VETERINARY SPECIFICS,

FOR THE CURE OF

## HORSES, CATTLE, SHEEP, HOGS AND DOGS.

---

The greatest improvement of the day is the treatment of sick ANIMALS by HOMEOPATHIC MEDICINES. All diseases of all kinds of Domestic Animals, Horses, Cattle, Sheep, Hogs and Dogs, as well as Poultry and Birds, are cured by Specific Homeopathic Veterinary Medicines with a promptness, certainty and ease truly astonishing.

Instead of the crude, unnatural means employed by the old school, the bottling, balling, drugging and villainous mixtures usually poured down the animals' throats, and which so often are sure to kill, if the disease fails, the owner gives a few drops of simple medicine on a bit of sugar or in water, without the least trouble—the medicine being as easily given to an ox as to a baby—and in a marvelous short time the disease is cured.

Experience proves that all diseases of domestic animals are perfectly controlled by the small doses and mild means of this system, and that horses and cattle are as readily cured as women and children.

The most inveterate and fatal diseases, which baffle the most energetic and skillful old school treatment, are cured like magic by these simple VETERINARY SPECIFICS. Cases of **Cough, Founder, Colic, Inflammation, Mange, Scratches, Distemper, Inflamed Eyes, Staggers,** and even **Spavin** and **Heaves,** are cured with a rapidity and certainty perfectly astonishing to those who have never witnessed the effects of these Specifics.

These Specifics not only save all trouble in giving medicine to animals, but restore and save a large proportion of animals otherwise lost or rendered valueless by disease. They are put up in *bottles of fluid*, containing each one hundred or more doses, and each case is accompanied with a *Book of Directions* and a small glass instrument—the Medicator—with which the proper dose is taken from the bottle and administered to the animal in the mouth or on the tongue, WITHOUT THE LEAST TROUBLE OR DELAY.

**The Manual of Directions** contains a full description of all diseases of horses, cattle, sheep, hogs and dogs, with full, particular directions for the treatment of each, so that any intelligent person may use them with success.

HUMPHREYS' HOMEOPATHIC VETERINARY SPECIFICS have been in use ELEVEN YEARS among all classes of people for the cure of sick horses, cattle, sheep, hogs and dogs, with the most wonderful success.

**Farmers and Agriculturists** use them, who raise and handle all kinds of domestic animals—careful, prudent, economical men, who know the value of all kinds of stock and the efficacy of all kinds of treatment, and who know how to value and appreciate an improvement.

**Importers and breeders** of blooded stock, who follow this as a business, and where the loss of a single animal involves the loss of hundreds or thousands of dollars.

**Livery-stable men,** and professional horse dealers and horse fanciers, all praise and use them.

**Traveling Menageries** and circus men, who own and have constantly hundreds of horses on the road, traveling over every part of the country, and who, using this system, rarely lose an animal, while those who use the old " drugging, balling and bottling " treatment lose thousands of dollars worth every year.

**Horse Railroads** in cities and large towns, who use hundreds of horses who always have sick horses on hand, and to whom the fees of veterinary doctors and losses of animals form a very large item of expense and loss—these use them extensively, and give them all praise.

---

WILLIAM LEWIS, agent of HOWE'S LONDON Circus, says:

"I have seen the effects of HUMPHREYS' HOMEOPATHIC VETERINARY SPECIFICS at Mehrbach's stables, in this city, and have used them myself with the best possible results, and would not be without them for any consideration. I shall do all I can to use and recommend them to my friends and acquaintances everywhere."

Read what JAMES H. WALLACE, of the Ninth Avenue Railroad Company, of New York City, and others, say of them:

"Mr. Wallace has charge of the horses of the Ninth Avenue Railroad Company, and has had as extensive experience in the care and treatment of horses as any man in New York, having been many years in his present business. He is thoroughly candid and reliable. He has the care of over three hundred horses, and for four years has used DR. HUMPHREYS' VETERINARY SPECIFICS in all cases of sickness occurring in the stables, and the general result is, that he has not **lost a horse by disease in these four years.** Some have been killed by accidents, broken legs, etc., but not one has died of disease. The average number of deaths by disease before commencing this treatment, and in other stables with the same number of horses, under other treatment, is from *two* to *three per month.* He has cured almost every disease to which the horse is subject, as there are always from three to twenty horses in the sick-bay. He has cured hundreds of cases of **Colic,** seldom requiring more than one or two doses, or more than a few minutes or an hour to cure a case. **Diarrhœas** rarely require the second dose of medicine. **Inflammations of the Head,** otherwise resulting in **Staggers,** are completely controlled in a few hours. **Lung Fevers** have repeatedly been cured in three or four days. They have had NINETEEN cases of **Pneumonia** during the season, and have cured every one of them with these Specifics. **Inflammation of the Bowels** has been cured in two or three days. Scores of cases of **Distemper** or **Strangles** have been cured. So of **Farcy. Founder** rarely occurs and is soon cured. The most violent cases of **Cough,** evidently bronchitis, have been cured in a few hours, and old cases of **Cough** and difficult breathing, or **Heaves,** have been cured. The remedies have perfect control over **Diseases of the Kidneys and Urinary Organs.** A horse coming in over-heated, during very hot weather, at once gets a few drops of the AA, and in an incredibly short space of time all danger of **Phrenitis, Staggers** or other disease has passed. So the list might be extended through every disease to which the horse is subject. These medicines have been almost invaluable, saving time, sickness, loss, and thousands of dollars of property every year."

Mr. Wallace will take pleasure in giving any gentleman further information.

Many persons who own but a single valuable horse or cow find it pays to use these VETERINARY SPECIFICS, and to own a case of them.

SAMUEL WHELPLEY is the Veterinary Superintendent of the New York Tenth Avenue Horse Railroad Company. He has five hundred and eighty horses in charge, and gives similar testimony.

ISAAC and SOLOMON MEERBACH, the well known extensive dealers in horses on Twenty-fourth street, New York, have been using these VETERINARY SPECIFICS for ten years or more past, and give them their unqualified recommendation. They use them extensively for all diseases among horses in their stables, and say that they *save thousands of dollars* every year by their use.

GEO. E. WARING, Esq., agricultural engineer, agricultural editor of the *New York Evening Post*, Ogden Farm, Newport, R. I. and author of the well-known Ogden Farm papers in the American Agriculturist, writes as follows:

"DEAR SIR—If my testimony can add to the public knowledge of the value of your HOMEOPATHIC VETERINARY SPECIFICS, I shall be glad. I regard your MANUAL of Veterinary Homeopathy as the only one that is sufficiently concise and clear for the comprehension of ordinary farmers, and since my acquaintance with it I have relied entirely upon your Veterinary Specifics in the treatment of my animals. The results have been uniformly good, save in one case in which I mistook the symptoms. I am impelled to write this as I have just cured a five hundred dollar Jersey cow of a severe attack of milk fever, by the use of your remedies alone."

The following gentlemen are also referred to who have purchased complete cases, and nearly all of whom have testified in terms similar to the foregoing:

Burdett Loomis, Windsor Locks, Conn.,
Samuel Campbell, Esq., New York, Mills, Utica, N. Y.,
Stephen Thorn, Esq., Thorndale, N. Y.,
A. Williamson, Bedford, N. Y.,
Peter W. Jones, Amherst, N. Y.,
Col. Amasa Sprague, Providence, R. I.,
E. W. Benjamin, Falls City, Neb.,
Chas. A. Kimball, Prop'r of Astor House Stables, N. Y.,
Rev'd Geo. F. Dickinson, New Springfield, New York,
Mr. Palmer, Sup't of Brooklyn City Horse Railroad,
N. P. Boyer & Co., Proprietors American Stock Journal, Parkesburg, Pa.,
C. W. Hurley & Co., Galveston, Texas,
Asterides Welch, Chestnut Hills, Pa.,
Dr. J. W. Weldon, Fordham, New York.,
Geo. Farnsworth, Homeopathic Veterinary Stables, 54th St. and Broadway, N. Y.,
Lewis A. White, 213 West 13th St., N. Y.,
John Briggs, Bedford, N. Y.,
Ed. Richardson, Auburn, N. Y.,
Austin H. Fisher, Adams, N. Y.,
A. Stohr, 296 Pavonia Ave., Jersey City
Mr. Coop, Manager of Barnum's Traveling Museum and Menagerie,
S. L. Smith, Cincinnati, O., Superintendent of City Horse R. R.,
Coblenz & Kaufman, Baltimore, Md.,
D. H. Smith, Sparta, Wis.,
F. B. McCanna, Pittsburgh, Pa.,
S. A. Viets, Springfield, Mass.

---

## LIST AND PRICES OF
# HUMPHREYS' HOMEOPATHIC VETERINARY SPECIFICS,
### And the more prominent Diseases and Conditions they are adapted to Cure.

**AA.—Cures Fevers,** Congestions or Inflammations; Lung Fever, Pneumonia, Inflammations of the Lungs or Bronchia, Head, Eyes, Throat or Belly; Quinsy, Staggers and Fits, Inflammation, Colic.

**BB.—Cures Results of Strains,** Injuries or Overwork; Founders, Laminitis, Rheumatism, Lameness, Blood or Incipient Bone Spavin or Curb, Stifle, etc.

**CC.—Cures Distemper,** Glanders, Farcy, Strangles, Swelled Glands in Horses, and Scab and Rot in Sheep.

**DD.—Cures Bots,** Worms or Grubs, Colic and disease in consequence of Worms.

**EE.—Cures all Diseases of the Air Passages,** Coughs, Influenza, Heaves, Broken or Thick Wind, Lung Fever, (in alternation with AA.,) Inflamed Lungs or Chest.

**FF.—Cures Colic,** Belly-ache, Hoven or Wind-blown, Diarrhœa, Dysentery, Liquid or Bloody Discharges.

**GG.—Prevents a threatened Miscarriage** or casting of Foal, or slinking of Calf, and assists cleansing after delivery.

**HH.—Cures all Urinary Complaints,** Strangury, Scanty, Suppressed or Bloody Urination, Inflamed Kidneys or Bladder, Urinary or Kidney Colic.

**II.—Cures Eruptive Diseases,** Mange, Farcy, Grease, Thrush, Abscess, Ulcers, Fistula, Swellings and Erysipelas.

**JJ.—Cures Jaundice** or Yellows, Bad Condition, Indigestion, Constipation, Staring Coat, Unthriftiness, Paralysis, either Spinal or of Single Parts.

## PRICE.

| | |
|---|---|
| Mahogany Case, complete, 10 bottles and Veterinary Manual | $10 00 |
| Single bottles | 1 00 |
| Veterinary Manual | 50 |
| Medicators | 35 |

N. B.—These Veterinary Medicines being fluid in glass bottles, cannot be sent by mail. But we will send a full case at $10, or even $5 worth, by express, *and pre-pay ourselves.* If only *one* or *two* bottles are ordered, the *purchaser must pay the express,* unless it is very near.

Sold by dealers or sent by express, as above. Address

Humphreys' Specific Homeopathic Medicine Co.,

562 Broadway, New York.

www.ingramcontent.com/pod-product-compliance
Lightning Source LLC
LaVergne TN
LVHW020127110826
845151LV00001B/294

* 9 7 8 1 4 2 5 5 4 0 7 3 9 *